Japanese Kampo Diet

Tony Salvitti

Copyright © 2014
Tony Salvitti

**Dedicated to:
Sensei Yamada
and
Sifu Kwan Li**

Two awesome men that took the time to pass on knowledge and skills. I am honored to have been the student of both amazing Masters!

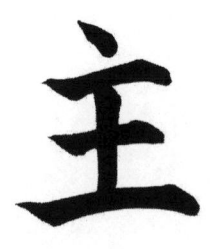

主

Contents

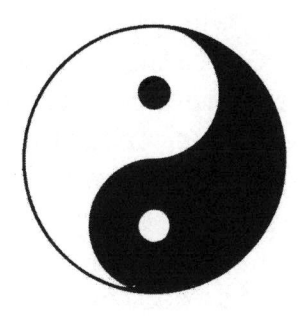

Origin of Kampo- 6

Kampo diet- 15

Kampo diagnosis methods- 60

Kampo herbs- 66

Kampo lifestyle- 104

Deer antler-Secret formula- 109

References- 131

Origin of Kampo

The use of herbs in itself or in combination with certain types of food in combinations has been around for thousands of years. As it is well known in ancient China was believed to have been first brought to Japan by way of Korea around the 5th or 6th Century A.D. By the beginning of 7th Century much information about Chinese medicine had reached Japan. It was not just medicine, Chinese traders also provided knowledge of Buddhism, and martial arts. It is largely because of this connection that during the Nara (710-794) and Heian (794-1192) periods, medicine was mainly provided by Buddhist Monks. By this time, the Chinese medical system was widely disseminated, soon becoming the standard medical system in Japan. The best example of how much medical knowledge was held by the ancient Japanese can be found by 808 A.D., the year that the Dido Rui Ju Howas published. Containing one hundred volumes of the most current medical knowledge, this work also contained various traditional therapeutic, or folk, remedies, well-known in the shrines and homes of Japan. This enormous compilation of medical knowledge was commissioned by Emperor Kanmu, based on his desire to retain the vast wealth of Japanese medical knowledge.

In 984 A.D., the Japanese physician Yasuyori Tamba wrote the Ishimpo (or Yi Xin Fang), which translates as 'The Essence of Medicine and Therapeutic Methods.' This text, the oldest surviving Japanese medical text, is a compilation of medical knowledge and theories that were prevalent during the Sui (589-618 A.D.) and the Tang Dynasties (618-907 A.D.). The Ishimpoquotes from hundreds of ancient Chinese medical texts, many of which had already been lost in China. It is largely because it was able to compile these dead texts that the Ishimpois so valued among scholars who study the medicinal history of the Sui and Tang Dynasties.

During the Edo period (16th to 18th century):

This Edo period became the distillation of all the Chinese medicine into the Japanese unique healing art Kampo, with the splitting of the two major styles of this therapeutic technique, each with different operating philosophies. The two schools were the Goseiha School (School of Later Developments in Medicine) and the Kohoha (School of Classical Formulas).

The Goseiha School was founded by Dosan Manase, who lived from 1507 to 1594. He was a student of Sanki Tashiro (1465-1537) and stayed in China for twelve years, spending his time there studying the medical systems used in the Jin (1115-1234 A.D.) and Yuan (1279-1368 A.D.) dynasties. There Manase found that the basis for Jin Yuan medicine was the dichotomy of the yin and the yang, as well as the **five elements** theories, which compared the human body to a small universe. Manase wrote many textbooks such as Keitekishu. He also established a medical school, Keitekiin and trained several hundred physicians. Manase's most significant contribution to Japanese medicine is also his most subtle; his ideas of simplicity and practicality, imparted through his lectures and his writing in Keitekishu, came to serve as a thematic foundation of the development of Kampo.

As the Jin Yuan style of medicine became to see wide practice in Japan, a small group of physicians began to criticize it. They claimed that it was ideology based only on speculative theory and they advocated a return to the classical concepts of Chinese medicine. They particularly advocated returning to the concepts and the teachings of the Shang Han Lun, translated as the 'Treatise on Cold Damage' and Jinkui Yaolue (Essential Prescriptions of the Golden Coffer). These texts were written over a thousand years earlier, and were hallmarks of the Kan period (Han Dynasty, 202 BC −220 A.D.). It is because these scholars sought a return to Kan medicine that they were, this group of physicians were referred to as Kohoha, or 'followers of the classic method.' The Kohoha School was proposed by Geni Nagoya, who lived from 1628 to 1696, then advocated by other proponents such as Konzan Goto (1659-1733), Toyou Yamawaki (1705-1762), and Todo Yoshimasu (1702-1773).

Todo Yoshimasu is considered to be one of the most influential figures in the history of Kampo medicine. Known for his positivistic Kampo approach, Yoshimasu was known as willing to accept and use any technique so long as it proved clinically effective, regardless of the surrounding theories or its particular philosophical background. Yoshimasu is most credited for his work in developing Kampo abdominal diagnosis. His abdominal diagnostic theories and practices not only became one of the most integral parts of today's Kampo, but they are also commonly credited with differentiating Kampo from traditional Chinese medicine. The many abdominal diagnoses were originally described in Chinese medical classics such as Shang Han Lun ('Treatise on Cold Damage') and Nan Jing ('Canon of Eighty-One Difficult Issues'), this specific method had long been abandoned in China.

During the later part of the Edo period, many Kampo practitioners integrated the two teachings, utilizing the strengths of both the Goseiha and Kohoha schools. They are known as disciples of the Sechu-ha, or 'eclectic' school of Japanese medicine.

Determining an appropriate Kampo formula requires a good diagnosis. **Sho** is a Kampo diagnosis based on a given patient's symptoms and patterns of disease.

Sho is far different from Western diagnoses. Patients with the same disease can have a totally different sho (disease/affliction) and be prescribed different Kampo prescriptions. This is unique to kampo, the same Kampo formulas may be used on patients with different diseases, if they have the same sho.

Each patient's sho is determined within the context of an Eastern view of human anatomy and physiology as well as illness.

Kampo uses a unique cognitive paradigm, making extensive use of tools such as:

- Yin and Yang,
- Exterior and Interior.
- Cold and Heat.
- Vascular (deficiency) and Repletion (excess).
- Five organs (heart, lungs, spleen, kidneys, and liver).
- Ki (ch'i, qi, prana, mana, ka, vital force).

Meiji Period (19th century):

The success of Kampo medicine is the fact that these healers were used not only for the common people, but also for Shoguns and emperors until the beginning of the Meiji period. As a side note, it is interesting to mention that during the middle years of the Edo period, European and American medicine was imported to Japan, and practiced as 'alternative' medicine. Despite its extraordinary popularity, Kampo medicine entered a period of rapid decline when the Meiji government decided to recognize only the German medical system, going with medicinal modernization sweeping the western world. By 1883, the Japanese government passed a law that retracted the medical licenses of any existing Kampo practitioners. Despite losing legal standing, a small number of these doctors continued to practice privately.

Showa Period (20th century):

During the middle of the Showa period, Kampo medicine began to regain its former popularity, while gaining increasingly international, recognition. Acupuncture, an integral part of Kampo medicine, saw a sharp increase in use. When the New York Times published an article about acupuncture. The practice of Kampo medicine also increased when Japan began to manufacture high-quality extracted herbal granules in 1957. Kampo medicine also saw an overall increase in popularity and usage when it was added to Japan's national health insurance plan in 1976.

Current Kampo usage in Japan:

In modern Japan, Kampo medicine has been fully legitimated and has been widely integrated into Japan's health care system.

An article on Kampo medicine published in the August 21, 1993 issue of the medical journal The Lancet reported that 70% of the 200,000 physicians in Japan regularly prescribe Kampo drugs to their patients. Of those types of physicians who regularly prescribe Kampo medicine and treatments, high percentages are found among gynecologists, with 88% prescribing Kampo medicines or techniques, followed by urologists (83%) and cardiologists (83%).

A survey conducted by Nikkei Medical indicated some of the main reasons why there has been an increase in the number of physicians prescribing Kampo medicine. This survey found that 65% of those physicians who had prescribed Kampo medicine believed that 'Western medicine has inherent limits' that could be compensated for by these forms of treatment. 32% answered that they might not have prescribed Kampo medicine in the past, but were swayed by the strong 'availability of scientific data' indicating the efficacy of Kampo. Finally, 31% offered that they only offered this medicine because of what they described as 'strong demand from patients.'

Kampo is currently covered by the Japanese national health insurance plan. At the present, 148 Kampo medicinal formulas are recognized by the Ministry of Health and the Ministry of Labor and Welfare, in addition to being covered by the National Health Insurance program.

Kampo diet

The kampo diet is an excellent way to gauge and keep your health in check. If you do this and exercise hopefully you will not need to even use kampo or other health care methods, because you will stay healthy.

Proper diet is very important for the recovery from many illnesses, as well as for the maintenance of good health. In fact, it is so important that diet has been deemed an integral part of Eastern medicine, food therapy. In Kampo, it is called Shokuyou, and in traditional Chinese medicine, this practice is known as Shi Liao.

In Western nutrition, the individual's approach will primarily focus on analyzing the nutritional values of each portion or meal. Kampo and traditional Chinese medicine, by contrast, emphasize the characteristics of whole foods, reflecting how they consider that every food has specific thermal characteristics, known as nature and flavor. Foods can be hot, warm, neutral, cool, or cold. Kampo practitioners consider these characteristics as elements that will affect an individual's constitution.

For example, a Western nutritionist may recommend a salad containing ingredients like lettuce, tomatoes, and oranges simply as a source of vitamins to a broad range of patients. According to the thermal nature of foods in Kampo, however, foods such as lettuce, tomatoes, and oranges are considered cold or cool. Thus, the over-consumption of such vegetables and fruits is not recommended for certain group of individuals (e.g., cold/spleen vacuity types). Conversely, if clients are expressing heat constitutional patterns, they may be encouraged to eat those foods that are cold or cool in nature. Ginger provides another interesting contrast. From a Western nutrition analysis point of view, ginger can be seen as simply a source of potassium. In Kampo, however, ginger is extremely valuable as both an herb and a medicinal food. The warming effect of ginger is highly valuable for patients with a cold constitution, and when combined with other herbs, it is able to enhance the effects of other warming herbs and decrease the undesirable side effects of herbs with cooling natures.

The main tenet of the Kampo diet is concept of balancing the Yin (cold) and the Yang (hot). For patients with a Yin constitution, it is recommended that they consume more Yang foods and minimize their intake of foods with a Yin nature.

For Yang patient the opposite is recommended: their doctor will recommend that they eat more Yin foods and decrease their intake of foods with a Yang nature. This balance is integral to understanding the Kampo diet. To simplify, when eating a meal one should note the **"cool-hot"** guide provided here and for example; If you were to have a all vegetable salad. The majority of the salad would be **cold-cool**. You need to balance this out with some food that is **warm-hot**. This could be a meat source such as beef, chicken, pork or turkey. Once you know the majority of foods that are **hot-warm** and **cold-cool**, the rest are **Neutral.** These can be combined with any food and complete your meal.

Dairy eggs

Food	Thermal Nature	Flavor
Butter	Cool	Sweet, fatty
Buttermilk	Cool	Sweet
Cheese	Neutral	Sweet, sour
Chicken egg	Neutral	Sweet
Cottage Cheese	Cool	Sweet, sour
Cream	Neutral	Sweet, fatty
Cream cheese	Cool	Sweet
Ghee	Neutral	Sweet, fatty
Margarine	Neutral	Sweet, fatty
Quail egg	Neutral	Sweet
Sour cream	Cool	Sour, sweet
Yogurt	Neutral	Sweet, sour

Fish & seafood

Food	Thermal Nature	Flavor
Abalone	Neutral	Sweet, salty
Amur catfish	Warm	Sweet
Asari clam	Cold	Sweet, salty
Basket clams	Cold	Sweet, salty
Bass	Neutral	Sweet, salty
Carp	Neutral	Sweet

Food	Thermal Nature	Flavor
Catfish	Neutral	Sweet
Caviar Fish	Cold	Salty
Turtle	Cool	Salty
Crab	Cold	Sweet, salty
Crayfish	Warm	Sweet, salty
Dojo Loach	Neutral	Sweet
Eel	Warm	Sweet
Hamaguri	Cold	Salty
Herring	Neutral	Sweet, salty
Mackerels	Warm	Sweet
Jellyfish	Neutral	Salty
Lobster	Neutral	Sweet, salty
Mackerel pike	Neutral	Sweet
Mussel	Warm	Salty
Octopus	Neutral	Sweet, salty
Olive flounder	Neutral	Sweet
Prawn	Warm	Sweet, salty
Puffer fish	Warm	Sweet
Salmon	Warm	Sweet
Sardine	Warm	Sweet, salty
Scallop	Neutral	Sweet
Sea breams	Neutral	Sweet
Sea Snail	Neutral	Sweet, salty
Sea urchins	Cool	Sweet, salty
Seabass	Neutral	Sweet
Shark	Neutral	Sweet, salty

Food	Thermal Nature	Flavor
Shark fin	Neutral	Sweet
Shrimp	Warm	Sweet
Skipjack tuna	Neutral	Sweet
Squid	Neutral	Salty, sweet
Sweetfish	Neutral	Sweet
Trout	Neutral	Sweet
Tuna	Warm	Sweet
Yellowtail	Warm	Sweet, sour

Fruits

Food	Thermal Nature	Flavor
Apple	Neutral	Sour, sweet
Apricot	Neutral	Sweet, sour
Avocado	Cool	Sweet
Banana	Cool	Sweet
Blackberry	Cool	Sweet, sour
Blackthorn	Cool	Sour
Blueberry	Cool	Sweet, sour
Carambola	Neutral	Sour, sweet
Cherry	Warm	Sweet
Cranberry	Cool	Sweet, sour
Currant, red	Cool	Sweet, sour
Dates	Neutral	Sweet
Fig	Neutral	Sweet
Ginko nuts	Neutral	Sweet, bitter
Goji Berry	Neutral	Sweet

Food	Thermal Nature	Flavor
Gooseberry	Cool	Sweat, sour
Grape	Neutral	Sweet, sour
Grapefruit	Cold	Sweet, sour
Guava	Warm	Sweet, astringent
Kiwi	Cold	Sweet, sour
Kumquat	Warm	Acrid, sweet, sour
Lemon	Cool	Sour, astringent
Longan	Warm	Sweet
Loquat	Neutral	Sweet, sour
Lychee	Warm	Sweet, sour
Mango	Cool	Sweet, sour
Melons	Cool	Sweet, aromatic
Mirabelle	Cool	Sweet, sour
Mulberry	Cool	Sweet, sour
Orange	Cool	Sweet, sour
Orange Peel	Warm	Sour, bitter, aromatic
Papaya	Neutral	Sweet, bitter
Passion	Cool	Bitter, bland
Peach	Warm	Sweet, sour
Pear	Cool	Sweet, sour
Persimmon	Cold	Sweet, astringent
Pineapple	Neutral	Sweet, astringent
Plum	Neutral	Sweet, sour
Pomegranate	Warm	Sweet, sour, astringent
Pomelo	Cool	Sweet, sour
Prune	Neutral	Sour, sweet
Quince	Cool	Bitter
Raspberry	Neutral	Sweet, sour

Food	Thermal Nature	Flavor
Star fruit	Cool	Sweet, sour
Strawberry	Cool	Sweet, sour
Tangerine	Cool	Sweet, sour
Ume Plum	Warm	Sour
Watermelon	Cold	Sweet

Beans & grains

Food	Thermal Nature	Flavor
Aduki bean	Neutral	Sweet, sour
Black Soybean	Neutral	Sweet
Black Turtle bean (Black bean)	Warm	Sweet
Chickpea (garbanzo bean)	Neutral	Sweet
Cowpea	Neutral	Sweet
Fava bean	Neutral	Sweet
Kidney bean	Neutral	Sweet
Lentil	Neutral	Sweet
Lima bean (butter bean)	Cool	Sweet
Mung bean (green bean, ryokuto)	Cool	Sweet
Natto	Warm	Sweet
Pea (green pea, endomame)	Neutral	Sweet
Soybean	Neutral	Sweet
String bean	Neutral	Sweet
Tofu	Cool	Sweet

Grains

Food	Thermal Nature	Flavor
Barley	Cool	Sweet, salty
Buckwheat	Cool	Sweet
Corn	Neutral	Sweet
Job's tears barley	Cool	Sweet, bland
Millet	Cool	Sweet, salty
Oats	Neutral	Sweet
Rice (non glutinous)	Neutral	Sweet
Rice, brown	Warm	Sweet
Rice, white	Warm	Sweet, bitter
Rye	Warm	Sweet, bitter
Spelt	Warm	Sweet
Wheat	Cool	Sweet
Wheat bran	Cool	Sweet
Wheat flour	Warm	Sweet

Nuts & seeds

Food	Thermal Nature	Flavor
Almond	Neutral	Sweet, bitter
Brazil nut	Neutral	Sweet, bitter
Cashew nut	Neutral	Sweet, fatty
Chestnut	Warm	Sweet
Coconut	Warm	Sweet
Flax seed	Neutral	Sweet, bland
Hazelnut	Neutral	Sweet, aromatic, slimy

Food	Thermal Nature	Flavor
Lotus seed	Neutral	Sweet, astringent
Peanut	Neutral	Sweet
Peanut butter	Neutral	Sweet, fatty
Pine nut	Warm	Sweet
Pistachio	Neutral	Sweet, bitter
Pumpkin seed	Warm	Sweet
Sesame	Neutral	Sweet
Sunflower	Neutral	Sweet
Walnut	Warm	Sweet

Vegetables & mushrooms

Food	Thermal Nature	Flavor
Alfalfa sprouts	Cool	Bitter
Artichoke	Cool	Bitter, sweet
Arugula	Cool	Acrid, bitter
Asparagus	Cold	Sweet, bitter
Bamboo Shoots	Cold	Sweet
Bay leaf	Warm	Acrid, bitter
Beet	Neutral	Sweet, bitter
Bitter melon	Cold	Sweet, bitter
Bok Choy	Cool	Sweet
Broccoli	Neutral	Sweet
Burdock root	Cool	Acrid, bitter
Cabbage	Neutral	Sweet, bitter
Carrot	Neutral	Sweet, acrid
Cauliflower	Neutral	Sweet, bitter

Food	Thermal Nature	Flavor
Celery	Cool	Sweet, bitter
Chard	Cool	Sweet, bitter
Chinese leek	Warm	Acrid
Chrysanthemum greens	Neutral	Acrid, sweet
Coriander	Warm	Acrid
Cucumber	Cold	Sweet, bitter
Dill	Warm	Acrid
Eggplant	Cool	Sweet
Endive	Cool	Bitter, sweet
Fuki	Warm	Bitter
Green pepper	Neutral	Acrid, sweet
Japanese parsley	Cool	Sweet
Kale	Neutral	Acrid, sweet
Kohlrabi	Neutral	Acrid, sweet, bitter
Konjac	Cool	Sweet
Leek	Warm	Acrid, sweet
Lettuce	Cool	Bitter, sweet
Lotus root	Neutral	Sweet, astringent
Lovage	Cool	Bitter, acrid
Mustard green	Warm	Acrid
Napa cabbage	Cool	Sweet
Okra	Neutral	Bitter, sweet, slimy
Olive	Neutral	Sweet, sour, astringent
Onion	Warm	Acrid, Sweet
Parsley	Warm	Acrid
Parsnip	Neutral	Sweet, bitter, acrid
Potato	Neutral	Sweet
Pumpkin	Warm	Sweet

Food	Thermal Nature	Flavor
Radish	Cool	Acrid, sweet
Rakkyo	Warm	Acrid, bitter
Rhubarb	Cold	Sour
Rhubarb root	Cold	Bitter
Sauerkraut	Cool	Sour
Scallion	Warm	Acrid
Shiso	Warm	Acrid
Sorrel	Cool	Sour
Soybean sprout	Cool	Sweet
Spinach	Cool	Sweet
Squash	Warm	Sweet
Sweet Potato	Neutral	Sweet
Taro (Satoimo)	Neutral	Acrid
Tomato	Cool	Sweet, sour
Turnip	Cool	Acrid, bitter
Water chestnut	Cool	Sweet, bland
Watercress	Cool	Acrid, bitter
Yamaimo	Neutral	Sweet
Zucchini	Cool	Sweet, bitter

Mushrooms

Food	Thermal Nature	Flavor
Jew's ear	Neutral	Sweet
Maitake	Warm	Sweet
Mushroom	Cool	Sweet, bland

```
Shiitake......Neutral      Sweet
Snow-fungus...Neutral      Sweet, bland
White fungus..Neutral      Sweet, bland
```

Seaweed

Type	Thermal Nature	Flavor
Agar (kanten)	Cold	Sweet
Hijiki	Cold	Salty
Irish Moss	Cool	Sweet, Salty
Kelp	Cold	Salty
Nori	Cold	Sweet, salty

Beverages (Non-alcoholic)

Type	Thermal Nature	Flavor
Black tea	Warm	Bitter, sweet, astringent.
Chamomile tea	Neutral	Bitter, sweet
Cocoa	Neutral	Sweet
Coffee Beverages	Warm	Bitter, acrid
Green tea	Cold	Bittersweet
Jasmine blossoms tea	Warm	Acrid
Milk (cow)	Neutral	Sweet
Milk (goat)	Warm	Sweet
Milk (human)	Neutral	Sweet, salty
Milk (sheep)	Warm	Sweet
Soy Milk	Neutral	Sweet
Uron Tea	Cool	Bitter, sweet, astringent

Beverages (Alcoholic)

Type	Thermal Nature	Flavor
Beer	Cool	Bitter, sweet
Red Wine	Warm	Bitter, acrid, sweet
Sake	Warm	Sweet, acrid, bitter
Shochu	Warm	Acrid, sweet
White wine	Cool	Sour, sweet

Spices and cooking herbs

Type	Thermal Nature	Flavor
Anise	Warm	Acrid, sweet
Basil	Warm	Acrid
Black Pepper	Hot	Acrid
Borage	Cool	Bitter, sweet, salty
Caraway seed	Warm	Acrid, sweet
Cardamom	Warm	Acrid, aromatic
Cayenne pepper	Hot	Acrid
Chervil	Cool	bitter, sweet
Cinnamon	Hot	Acrid, sweet
Clove	Warm	Acrid
Cumin	Warm	Acrid, sweet
Curry	Warm	Acrid, bitter
Fennel	Warm	Acrid
Fenugreek	Warm	Bitter, acrid
Garlic	Warm	Acrid
Ginger	Warm	Acrid

Type	Thermal Nature	Flavor
Horserasdish	Warm	Acrid
Juniper berry	Warm	Acrid, bitter
Lavender	Cool	Bitter, acrid
Licorice	Neutral	Sweet, bitter
Marjoram	Cool	Acrid
Mint	Cool	Acrid
Mugwort	Warm	Bitter, acrid
Mustard	Warm	Acrid, bitter
Mustard Seeds	Warm	Acrid
Myoga ginger	Cold	Bitter, sweet

Type	Thermal Nature	Flavor
Nutmeg	Warm	Acrid
Oregano	Neutral	Acrid, bitter
Paprika	Warm	Bitter, sweet
Pepper, white	Hot	Acrid
Peppermint	Cool	Acrid
Rosemary	Warm	Acrid
Saffron	Warm	Sweet, Acrid
Sage	Warm	Bitter, acrid
Salt	Cold	Salty
Sichuan pepper	Hot	Acrid
Spearmint	Warm	Acrid
Star aniseed	Warm	Acrid, sweet
Tarragon	Warm	Bittter, acrid
Thyme	Warm	Acrid
Turmeric	Warm	Acrid, bitter
Wasabi	Warm	Acrid

Acrid foods

Type	Thermal Nature	Flavor
Red Wine	Warm	Bitter, acrid, sweet
Sake	Warm	Sweet, acrid, bitter
Shochu	Warm	Acrid, sweet
Coffee	Warm	Bitter, acrid
Jasmine tea	Warm	Acrid
Cheese (goat's milk)	Warm	Acrid, salty, sweet
Cheese (sheep's milk)	Warm	Acrid, salty, sweet
Kumquat (kinkan)	Warm	Acrid, sweet, sour
Horse Meat	Cool	Acrid, bitter
Cider Vinegar	Neutral	Sour, acrid
Soybean oil	Warm	Acrid, sweet
Lavender	Cool	Bitter, acrid
Marjoram	Cool	Acrid
Mint	Cool	Acrid
Peppermint	Cool	Acrid
Black Pepper	Hot	Acrid
Cayenne pepper	Hot	Acrid
Cinnamon	Hot	Acrid, sweet
Pepper, white	Hot	Acrid
Sichuan pepper	Hot	Acrid
Oregano	Neutral	Acrid, bitter
Anise	Warm	Acrid, sweet
Basil	Warm	Acrid
Caraway seed	Warm	Acrid, sweet
Cardamom	Warm	Acrid, aromatic
Clove	Warm	Acrid

Type	Thermal Nature	Flavor
Cumin	Warm	Acrid, sweet
Curry	Warm	Acrid, bitter
Fennel	Warm	Acrid
Fenugreek seed	Warm	Bitter, acrid
Garlic	Warm	Acrid
Ginger	Warm	Acrid
Horserasdish	Warm	Acrid
Juniper berry	Warm	Acrid, bitter
Mugwort (yomogi)	Warm	Bitter, acrid
Mustard	Warm	Acrid, bitter
Mustard Seeds	Warm	Acrid
Nutmeg	Warm	Acrid
Rosemary	Warm	Acrid
Saffron	Warm	Sweet, Acrid
Sage	Warm	Bitter, acrid
Spearmint	Warm	Acrid
Star aniseed	Warm	Acrid, sweet
Tarragon	Warm	Bitter, acrid
Thyme	Warm	Acrid
Turmeric	Warm	Acrid, bitter
Wasabi	Warm	Acrid
Watercress	Cool	Acrid, bitter
Coriander	Warm	Acrid
Dill	Warm	Acrid
Arugula	Cool	Acrid, bitter
Burdock root	Cool	Acrid, bitter
Lovage	Cool	Bitter, acrid
Radish	Cool	Acrid, sweet

Type	Thermal Nature	Flavor
Turnip	Cool	Acrid, bitter
Carrot	Neutral	Sweet, acrid
Chrysanthemum	Neutral	Acrid, sweet
Green pepper	Neutral	Acrid, sweet
Kale	Neutral	Acrid, sweet
Kohlrabi	Neutral	Acrid, sweet, bitter
Parsnip	Neutral	Sweet, bitter, acrid
Taro	Neutral	Acrid
Bay leaf	Warm	Acrid, bitter
Chinese leek	Warm	Acrid
Leek	Warm	Acrid, sweet
Mustard green	Warm	Acrid
Onion	Warm	Acrid, Sweet
Parsley	Warm	Acrid
Rakkyo	Warm	Acrid, bitter
Scallion	Warm	Acrid
Shiso	Warm	Acrid

Bitter foods

Type	Thermal Nature	Flavor
Beer	Cool	Bitter, sweet
Red Wine	Warm	Bitter, acrid, sweet
Sake	Warm	Sweet, acrid, bitter
Green tea	Cold	Bitter, sweet, astringent
Uron Tea	Cool	Bitter, sweet, astringent
Chamomile tea	Neutral	Bitter, sweet

Type	Thermal Nature	Flavor
Black tea	Warm	Bitter, sweet, astringent.
Coffee	Warm	Bitter, acrid
Passion fruit	Cool	Bitter, bland
Quince Fruits	Cool	Bitter
Ginko nuts	Neutral	Sweet, bitter
Papaya Fruits	Neutral	Sweet, bitter
Orange Peel	Warm	Sour, bitter, aromatic
Rice, glutinous	Warm	Sweet, bitter
Rye	Warm	Sweet, bitter
Horse Meat	Cool	Acrid, bitter
Almond Nuts	Neutral	Sweet, bitter
Brazil nut	Neutral	Sweet, bitter
Pistachio	Neutral	Sweet, bitter
Myoga ginger	Cold	Bitter, sweet
Borage	Cool	Bitter, sweet, salty
Chervil	Cool	bitter, sweet
Lavender	Cool	Bitter, acrid
Licorice	Neutral	Sweet, bitter
Oregano	Neutral	Acrid, bitter
Curry	Warm	Acrid, bitter
Fenugreek	Warm	Bitter, acrid
Juniper berry	Warm	Acrid, bitter
Mugwort	Warm	Bitter, acrid
Mustard	Warm	Acrid, bitter
Paprika	Warm	Bitter, sweet
Sage	Warm	Bitter, acrid
Tarragon	Warm	Bittter, acrid
Turmeric	Warm	Acrid, bitter

Type	Thermal Nature	Flavor
Watercress	Cool	Acrid, bitter
Asparagus	Cold	Sweet, bitter
Bitter melon	Cold	Sweet, bitter
Cucumber	Cold	Sweet, bitter
Rhubarb root	Cold	Bitter
Alfalfa sprouts	Cool	Bitter
Artichoke	Cool	Bitter, sweet
Arugula	Cool	Acrid, bitter
Burdock root	Cool	Acrid, bitter
Celery	Cool	Sweet, bitter
Chard	Cool	Sweet, bitter
Endive	Cool	Bitter, sweet
Lettuce	Cool	Bitter, sweet
Lovage	Cool	Bitter, acrid
Turnip	Cool	Acrid, bitter
Zucchini	Cool	Sweet, bitter
Beet	Neutral	Sweet, bitter
Cabbage	Neutral	Sweet, bitter
Cauliflower	Neutral	Sweet, bitter
Kohlrabi	Neutral	Acrid, sweet, bitter
Okra	Neutral	Bitter, sweet, slimy
Parsnip	Neutral	Sweet, bitter, acrid
Bay leaf	Warm	Acrid, bitter
Fuki	Warm	Bitter
Rakkyo	Warm	Acrid, bitter

Salty foods

Type	Thermal Nature	Flavor
Milk (human)	Neutral	Sweet, salty
Cheese	Warm	Acrid, salty, sweet
Asari clam	Cold	Sweet, salty
Basket clams	Cold	Sweet, salty
Caviar	Cold	Salty
Crab	Cold	Sweet, salty
Hamaguri	Cold	Salty
Turtle	Cool	Salty
Sea urchins	Cool	Sweet, salty
Abalone	Neutral	Sweet, salty
Bass	Neutral	Sweet, salty
Herring	Neutral	Sweet, salty
Jellyfish	Neutral	Salty
Lobster	Neutral	Sweet, salty
Octopus	Neutral	Sweet, salty
Oyster	Neutral	Sweet, salty
Sea Snail	Neutral	Sweet, salty
Shark	Neutral	Sweet, salty
Squid	Neutral	Salty, sweet
Crayfish	Warm	Sweet, salty
Mussel	Warm	Salty
Prawn	Warm	Sweet, salty
Sardine	Warm	Sweet, salty
Miso	Cold	Salty
Soy sauce	Cool	Salty
Barley	Cool	Sweet, salty

Type	Thermal Nature	Flavor
Millet	Cool	Sweet, salty
Beef kidney	Neutral	Salty
Pork	Neutral	Sweet, salty
Hijiki	Cold	Salty
Kelp	Cold	Salty
Nori	Cold	Sweet, salty
Irish Moss	Cool	Sweet, Salty
Salt	Cold	Salty
Borage	Cool	Bitter, sweet, salty

Sweet foods

Type	Thermal Nature	Flavor
Beer	Cool	Bitter, sweet
White wine	Cool	Sour, sweet
Red Wine	Warm	Bitter, acrid, sweet
Sake	Warm	Sweet, acrid, bitter
Shochu	Warm	Acrid, sweet
Green tea	Cold	Bitter, sweet, astringent
Uron Tea	Cool	Bitter, sweet, astringent
Chamomile	Neutral	Bitter, sweet
Cocoa	Neutral	Sweet
Milk	Neutral	Sweet
Soy Milk	Neutral	Sweet
Black tea	Warm	Bitter, sweet, astringent.
Milk (goat)	Warm	Sweet
Milk (sheep)	Warm	Sweet

Type	Thermal Nature	Flavor
Butter	Cool	Sweet, fatty
Buttermilk	Cool	Sweet
Cottage Cheese	Cool	Sweet, sour
Cream cheese	Cool	Sweet
Sour cream	Cool	Sour, sweet
Cheese	Neutral	Sweet, sour
Chicken egg	Neutral	Sweet
Cream	Neutral	Sweet, fatty
Ghee	Neutral	Sweet, fatty
Margarine	Neutral	Sweet, fatty
Quail egg	Neutral	Sweet
Yogurt	Neutral	Sweet, sour
Cheese	Warm	Acrid, salty, sweet
Asari clam	Cold	Sweet, salty
Basket clams	Cold	Sweet, salty
Crab	Cold	Sweet, salty
Sea urchins	Cool	Sweet, salty
Abalone	Neutral	Sweet, salty
Bass	Neutral	Sweet, salty
Carp	Neutral	Sweet
Dojo Loach	Neutral	Sweet
Herring	Neutral	Sweet, salty
Lobster	Neutral	Sweet, salty
Mackerel	Neutral	Sweet
Octopus	Neutral	Sweet, salty
Olive flounder	Neutral	Sweet
Oyster	Neutral	Sweet, salty
Scallop	Neutral	Sweet

Type	Thermal Nature	Flavor
Sea breams	Neutral	Sweet
Sea Snail	Neutral	Sweet, salty
Seabass	Neutral	Sweet
Shark	Neutral	Sweet, salty
Shark fin	Neutral	Sweet
Tuna	Neutral	Sweet
Squid	Neutral	Salty, sweet
Sweetfish	Neutral	Sweet
Trout	Neutral	Sweet
Catfish	Warm	Sweet
Crayfish	Warm	Sweet, salty
Eel	Warm	Sweet
Mackerel	Warm	Sweet
Prawn	Warm	Sweet, salty
Puffer fish	Warm	Sweet
Salmon	Warm	Sweet
Sardine	Warm	Sweet, salty
Shrimp	Warm	Sweet
Tuna	Warm	Sweet
Yellowtail	Warm	Sweet, sour
Honey	Neutral	Sweet
Sugar	Neutral	Sweet
Malt syrup	Warm	Sweet
Molasses	Warm	Sweet
Sugar	Warm	Sweet
Vanilla	Warm	Sweet
Grapefruit	Cold	Sweet, sour
Kiwi	Cold	Sweet, sour

Type	Thermal Nature	Flavor
Persimmon	Cold	Sweet, astringent
Watermelon	Cold	Sweet
Avocado	Cool	Sweet
Banana	Cool	Sweet
Blackberry	Cool	Sweet, sour
Blueberry	Cool	Sweet, sour
Cranberry	Cool	Sweet, sour
Currants	Cool	Sweet, sour
Mango	Cool	Sweet, sour
Melons	Cool	Sweet, aromatic
Mirabelle	Cool	Sweet, sour
Mulberry	Cool	Sweet, sour
Orange	Cool	Sweet, sour
Pear	Cool	Sweet, sour
Pomelo	Cool	Sweet, sour
Star fruit	Cool	Sweet, sour
Strawberry	Cool	Sweet, sour
Tangerine	Cool	Sweet, sour
Apple	Neutral	Sour, sweet
Apricot	Neutral	Sweet, sour
Carambola	Neutral	Sour, sweet
Dates	Neutral	Sweet
Fig	Neutral	Sweet
Ginko nuts	Neutral	Sweet, bitter
Goji Berry	Neutral	Sweet
Grape	Neutral	Sweet, sour
Loquat	Neutral	Sweet, sour
Papaya	Neutral	Sweet, bitter

Type	Thermal Nature	Flavor
Pineapple	Neutral	Sweet, astringent
Plum	Neutral	Sweet, sour
Prune	Neutral	Sour, sweet
Raspberry	Neutral	Sweet, sour
Cherry	Warm	Sweet
Guava	Warm	Sweet, astringent
Kumquat	Warm	Acrid, sweet, sour
Longan	Warm	Sweet
Lychee	Warm	Sweet, sour
Peach	Warm	Sweet, sour
Pomegranate	Warm	Sweet, sour, astringent
Barley	Cool	Sweet, salty
Buckwheat	Cool	Sweet
Job's tears	Cool	Sweet, bland
Millet	Cool	Sweet, salty
Wheat	Cool	Sweet
Wheat bran	Cool	Sweet
Corn	Neutral	Sweet
Oats	Neutral	Sweet
Rice	Neutral	Sweet
Rice, brown	Warm	Sweet
Rice, (ozo)	Warm	Sweet, bitter
Rye	Warm	Sweet, bitter
Wheat flour	Warm	Sweet
Spelt	Warm	Sweet
Lima bean	Cool	Sweet
Mung bean	Cool	Sweet
Tofu	Cool	Sweet

Type	Thermal Nature	Flavor
Aduki bean	Neutral	Sweet, sour
Black Soybean	Neutral	Sweet
Chickpea	Neutral	Sweet
Cowpea	Neutral	Sweet
Fava bean	Neutral	Sweet
Kidney bean	Neutral	Sweet
Lentil	Neutral	Sweet
Pea	Neutral	Sweet
Soybean	Neutral	Sweet
String bean	Neutral	Sweet
Black bean	Warm	Sweet
Natto	Warm	Sweet
Duck	Cool	Sweet
Frog	Cool	Sweet
Lamb	Hot	Sweet
Beef liver	Neutral	Sweet
Goose	Neutral	Sweet
Lard, pork	Neutral	sweet, fatty
Pork	Neutral	Sweet, salty
Quail	Neutral	Sweet
Rabbit	Neutral	Sweet
Veal	Neutral	Sweet
Beef	Warm	Sweet
Bone-marrow	Warm	Sweet, fattty
Chicken	Warm	Sweet
Goat meat	Warm	Sweet
Pheasant	Warm	Sweet, sour
Turkey	Warm	Sweet

Type	Thermal Nature	Flavor
Venison	Warm	Sweet
Wild boar	Warm	Sweet
Mushroom	Neutral	Sweet, bland
Jew's ear	Neutral	Sweet
Lion's Mane Mushroom	Neutral	Sweet
Oyster mushroom	Neutral	Sweet
Shiitake	Neutral	Sweet
Snow fungus	Neutral	Sweet, bland
White fungus	Neutral	Sweet, bland
Maitake	Warm	Sweet
Almond	Neutral	Sweet, bitter
Brazil nut	Neutral	Sweet, bitter
Cashew nut	Neutral	Sweet, fatty
Flax seed	Neutral	Sweet, bland
Hazelnut	Neutral	Sweet, aromatic, slimy
Lotus seed	Neutral	Sweet, astringent
Peanut Nuts	Neutral	Sweet
Peanut butter	Neutral	Sweet, fatty
Pistachio	Neutral	Sweet, bitter
Sesame	Neutral	Sweet
Sunflower	Neutral	Sweet
Chestnut	Warm	Sweet
Coconut	Warm	Sweet
Pine nut	Warm	Sweet
Pumpkin seed	Warm	Sweet
Walnut	Warm	Sweet
Olive Oil	Cool	Sweet, fatty
Corn oil	Neutral	Sweet

Type	Thermal Nature	Flavor
Peanut oil	Neutral	Sweet, fatty
Sesame oil	Neutral	Sweet, fatty
Sunflower oil	Neutral	Sweet, fatty
Canola oil	Warm	Sweet, fatty
Soybean oil	Warm	Acrid, sweet
Walnut oil	Warm	Sweet, fatty
Agar	Cold	Sweet
Nori	Cold	Sweet, salty
Irish Moss	Cool	Sweet, Salty
Myoga ginger	Cold	Bitter, sweet
Borage	Cool	Bitter, sweet, salty
Chervil	Cool	Bitter, sweet
Cinnamon	Hot	Acrid, sweet
Licorice	Neutral	Sweet, bitter
Anise	Warm	Acrid, sweet
Caraway seed	Warm	Acrid, sweet
Cumin	Warm	Acrid, sweet
Paprika	Warm	Bitter, sweet
Saffron	Warm	Sweet, Acrid
Star aniseed	Warm	Acrid, sweet
Water chestnut	Cool	Sweet, bland
Potato	Neutral	Sweet
Asparagus	Cold	Sweet, bitter
Bamboo Shoots	Cold	Sweet
Bitter melon	Cold	Sweet, bitter
Cucumber	Cold	Sweet, bitter
Artichoke	Cool	Bitter, sweet
Bok Choy	Cool	Sweet

Type	Thermal Nature	Flavor
Celery	Cool	Sweet, bitter
Chard	Cool	Sweet, bitter
Eggplant	Cool	Sweet
Endive	Cool	Bitter, sweet
Parsley	Cool	Sweet
Konjac	Cool	Sweet
Lettuce	Cool	Bitter, sweet
Napa cabbage	Cool	Sweet
Radish	Cool	Acrid, sweet
Soybean	Cool	Sweet
Spinach	Cool	Sweet
Tomato	Cool	Sweet, sour
Zucchini	Cool	Sweet, bitter
Beet	Neutral	Sweet, bitter
Broccoli	Neutral	Sweet
Cabbage	Neutral	Sweet, bitter
Carrot	Neutral	Sweet, acrid
Cauliflower	Neutral	Sweet, bitter
Green pepper	Neutral	Acrid, sweet
Kale	Neutral	Acrid, sweet
Kohlrabi	Neutral	Acrid, sweet, bitter
Lotus root	Neutral	Sweet, astringent
Okra	Neutral	Bitter, sweet, slimy
Olive	Neutral	Sweet, sour, astringent
Parsnip	Neutral	Sweet, bitter, acrid
Sweet Potato	Neutral	Sweet

Type	Thermal Nature	Flavor
Leek	Warm	Acrid, sweet
Onion	Warm	Acrid, Sweet
Pumpkin	Warm	Sweet
Squash	Warm	Sweet

Sour foods

Type	Thermal Nature	Flavor
White wine	Cool	Sour, sweet
Cottage Cheese	Cool	Sweet, sour
Sour cream	Cool	Sour, sweet
Cheese	Neutral	Sweet, sour
Yogurt	Neutral	Sweet, sour
Yellowtail	Warm	Sweet, sour
Grapefruit	Cold	Sweet, sour
Kiwi	Cold	Sweet, sour
Blackberry	Cool	Sweet, sour
Blackthorn	Cool	Sour
Blueberry	Cool	Sweet, sour
Cranberry	Cool	Sweet, sour
Currant, red	Cool	Sweet, sour
Gooseberry	Cool	Sweat, sour
Lemon	Cool	Sour, astringent
Mango	Cool	Sweet, sour
Mirabelle	Cool	Sweet, sour
Mulberry	Cool	Sweet, sour
Orange	Cool	Sweet, sour

Type	Thermal Nature	Flavor
Pear	Cool	Sweet, sour
Pomelo	Cool	Sweet, sour
Star fruit	Cool	Sweet, sour
Strawberry	Cool	Sweet, sour
Tangerine	Cool	Sweet, sour
Apple	Neutral	Sour, sweet
Apricot	Neutral	Sweet, sour
Carambola	Neutral	Sour, sweet
Grape	Neutral	Sweet, sour
Loquat	Neutral	Sweet, sour
Plum	Neutral	Sweet, sour
Prune	Neutral	Sour, sweet
Raspberry	Neutral	Sweet, sour
Kumquat	Warm	Acrid, sweet, sour
Lychee	Warm	Sweet, sour
Orange Peel	Warm	Sour, bitter, aromatic
Peach	Warm	Sweet, sour
Pomegranate	Warm	Sweet, sour, astringent
Ume Plum	Warm	Sour
Aduki bean	Neutral	Sweet, sour
Pheasant	Warm	Sweet, sour
Wheat vinegar	Cool	Sour
Cider Vinegar	Neutral	Sour, acrid
Red wine vinegar	Warm	Sour
Rice vinegar	Warm	Sour
Sherry Vinegar	Warm	Sour
Rhubarb	Cold	Sour
Sauerkraut	Cool	Sour

Type	Thermal Nature	Flavor
Sorrel	Cool	Sour
Tomato	Cool	Sweet, sour
Olive	Neutral	Sweet, sour, astringent

Hot foods

Type	Thermal Nature	Flavor
Lamb	Hot	Sweet
Black Pepper	Hot	Acrid
Cayenne pepper	Hot	Acrid
Cinnamon	Hot	Acrid, sweet
Pepper	Hot	Acrid
Sichuan pepper	Hot	Acrid

Warm foods

Type	Thermal Nature	Flavor
Red Wine	Warm	Bitter, acrid, sweet
Sake	Warm	Sweet, acrid, bitter
Shochu	Warm	Acrid, sweet
Black tea	Warm	Bittersweet
Coffee	Warm	Bitter, acrid
Jasmine tea	Warm	Acrid
Milk	Warm	Sweet
Cheese	Warm	Acrid, salty, sweet

Type	Thermal Nature	Flavor
Amur catfish	Warm	Sweet
Crayfish	Warm	Sweet, salty
Eel	Warm	Sweet
Jack mackerels	Warm	Sweet
Mussel	Warm	Salty
Prawn	Warm	Sweet, salty
Puffer fish	Warm	Sweet
Salmon	Warm	Sweet
Sardine	Warm	Sweet, salty
Shrimp	Warm	Sweet
Tuna	Warm	Sweet
Yellowtail	Warm	Sweet, sour
Malt syrup	Warm	Sweet
Molasses	Warm	Sweet
Sugar (brown)	Warm	Sweet
Vanilla	Warm	Sweet
Cherry	Warm	Sweet
Guava	Warm	Sweet, astringent
Kumquat	Warm	Acrid, sweet, sour
Longan	Warm	Sweet
Lychee	Warm	Sweet, sour
Orange	Warm	Sour, bitter, aromatic
Peach	Warm	Sweet, sour
Pomegranate	Warm	Sweet, sour, astringent
Ume Plum	Warm	Sour
Rice, brown	Warm	Sweet

Type	Thermal Nature	Flavor
Rice, white	Warm	Sweet, bitter
Rye	Warm	Sweet, bitter
Spelt	Warm	Sweet
Wheat flour	Warm	Sweet
Black beans	Warm	Sweet
Natto bean	Warm	Sweet
Beef	Warm	Sweet
Bone-marrow	Warm	Sweet, fatty
Chicken	Warm	Sweet
Goat	Warm	Sweet
Pheasant	Warm	Sweet, Sour
Turkey	Warm	Sweet
Venison	Warm	Sweet
Wild boar	Warm	Sweet
Maitake	Warm	Sweet
Anise	Warm	Sweet
Chestnut	Warm	Sweet
Coconut	Warm	Sweet
Pine nut	Warm	Sweet
Pumpkin seed	Warm	Sweet
Walnut Nuts	Warm	Sweet
Canola oil	Warm	Sweet, fatty
Red wine vinegar	Warm	Sweet
Rice vinegar	Warm	Sour
Sherry Vinegar	Warm	Sour
Soybean oil	Warm	Acrid, sour
Walnut oil	Warm	Sweet, acrid

Type	Thermal Nature	Flavor
Basil Spices	Warm	Acrid
Caraway seed	Warm	Acrid, sweet
Cardamom	Warm	Acrid, aromatic
Clove	Warm	Acrid
Cumin	Warm	Acrid, sweet
Curry	Warm	Acrid, bitter
Fennel	Warm	Acrid
Fenugreek seed	Warm	Bitter, acrid
Garlic	Warm	Acrid
Ginger	Warm	Acrid
Horseradish	Warm	Acrid
Juniper berry	Warm	Acrid, bitter
Mugwort	Warm	Bitter, acrid
Mustard	Warm	Acrid, bitter
Mustard Seeds	Warm	Acrid
Nutmeg	Warm	Acrid
Paprika	Warm	Bitter, sweet
Rosemary	Warm	Acrid
Saffron	Warm	Sweet, Acrid
Sage	Warm	Bitter, acrid
Spearmint	Warm	Acrid
Star aniseed	Warm	Acrid, sweet
Tarragon	Warm	Bitter, acrid
Thyme	Warm	Acrid
Turmeric	Warm	Acrid, bitter
Wasabi	Warm	Acrid
Coriander	Warm	Acrid
Dill	Warm	Acrid

Type	Thermal Nature	Flavor
Bay leaf	Warm	Acrid, bitter
Chinese leek	Warm	Acrid
Fuki	Warm	Bitter
Leek	Warm	Acrid, sweet
Mustard green	Warm	Acrid
Onion	Warm	Acrid, Sweet
Parsley	Warm	Acrid
Pumpkin	Warm	Sweet
Rakkyo	Warm	Acrid, bitter
Scallion	Warm	Acrid
Shiso	Warm	Acrid
Squash	Warm	Sweet

Bland or neutral foods

Type	Thermal Nature	Flavor
Chamomile tea	Neutral	Bitter, sweet
Cocoa	Neutral	Sweet
Milk	Neutral	Sweet
Milk (human)	Neutral	Sweet, salty
Soy Milk	Neutral	Sweet
Chicken egg	Neutral	Sweet
Cream	Neutral	Sweet, fatty
Ghee	Neutral	Sweet, fatty
Margarine	Neutral	Sweet, fatty
Quail egg	Neutral	Sweet
Yogurt Dairy	Neutral	Sweet, sour

Type	Thermal Nature	Flavor
Abalone	Neutral	Sweet, salty
Bass	Neutral	Sweet, salty
Carp	Neutral	Sweet
Catfish	Neutral	Sweet
Dojo Loach	Neutral	Sweet
Herring	Neutral	Sweet, salty
Jellyfish	Neutral	Salty
Lobster	Neutral	Sweet, salty
Mackerel	Neutral	Sweet
Mackerel pike	Neutral	Sweet
Octopus	Neutral	Sweet, salty
Olive flounder	Neutral	Sweet
Oyster	Neutral	Sweet, salty
Scallop	Neutral	Sweet
Sea breams	Neutral	Sweet
Sea Snail	Neutral	Sweet, salty
Seabass	Neutral	Sweet
Shark	Neutral	Sweet, salty
Shark fin	Neutral	Sweet
Skipjack tuna	Neutral	Sweet
Squid	Neutral	Salty, sweet
Sweetfish	Neutral	Sweet
Trout	Neutral	Sweet
Honey	Neutral	Sweet
Sugar (white)	Neutral	Sweet
Apple	Neutral	Sour, sweet
Apricot	Neutral	Sweet, sour
Carambola	Neutral	Sour, sweet

Type	Thermal Nature	Flavor
Dates	Neutral	Sweet
Fig	Neutral	Sweet
Ginko	Neutral	Sweet, bitter
Goji Berry	Neutral	Sweet
Grape	Neutral	Sweet, sour
Loquat	Neutral	Sweet, sour
Papaya	Neutral	Sweet, bitter
Pineapple	Neutral	Sweet, astringent
Plum	Neutral	Sweet, sour
Prune	Neutral	Sour, sweet
Raspberry	Neutral	Sweet, sour
Corn	Neutral	Sweet
Oats	Neutral	Sweet
Rice	Neutral	Sweet
Aduki bean	Neutral	Sweet, sour
Black Soybean	Neutral	Sweet
Chickpea	Neutral	Sweet
Cowpea	Neutral	Sweet
Fava bean	Neutral	Sweet
Kidney bean	Neutral	Sweet
Lentil	Neutral	Sweet
Pea	Neutral	Sweet
Soybean	Neutral	Sweet
String bean	Neutral	Sweet
Beef kidney	Neutral	Salty
Beef liver	Neutral	Sweet
Goose	Neutral	Sweet
Lard, pork	Neutral	Sweet, fatty

Type	Thermal Nature	Flavor
Pork	Neutral	Sweet, salty
Quail	Neutral	Sweet
Rabbit	Neutral	Sweet
Veal	Neutral	Sweet
Jew's ear	Neutral	Sweet
Oyster mushroom	Neutral	Sweet
Shiitake	Neutral	Sweet
Snow fungus	Neutral	Sweet, bland
White fungus	Neutral	Sweet, bland
Almond	Neutral	Sweet, bitter
Brazil	Neutral	Sweet, bitter
Cashew	Neutral	Sweet, fatty
Flax seed	Neutral	Sweet, bland
Hazelnut	Neutral	Sweet, aromatic, slimy
Lotus seed	Neutral	Sweet, astringent
Peanut	Neutral	Sweet
Peanut butter	Neutral	Sweet, fatty
Pistachio	Neutral	Sweet, bitter
Sesame	Neutral	Sweet
Sunflower Seed	Neutral	Sweet
Cider Vinegar	Neutral	Sour, acrid
Corn oil	Neutral	Sweet
Peanut oil	Neutral	Sweet, fatty
Sesame oil	Neutral	Sweet, fatty
Sunflower oil	Neutral	Sweet, fatty
Licorice	Neutral	Sweet, bitter
Oregano	Neutral	Acrid, bitter
Potato	Neutral	Sweet

Type	Thermal Nature	Flavor
Beet	Neutral	Sweet, bitter
Broccoli	Neutral	Sweet
Cabbage	Neutral	Sweet, bitter
Carrot	Neutral	Sweet, acrid
Cauliflower	Neutral	Sweet, bitter
Chrysanthemum	Neutral	Acrid, sweet
Green pepper	Neutral	Acrid, sweet
Kale	Neutral	Acrid, sweet
Kohlrabi	Neutral	Acrid, sweet, bitter
Lotus root	Neutral	Sweet, astringent
Okra	Neutral	Bitter, sweet, slimy
Olive	Neutral	Sweet, sour, astringent
Parsnip	Neutral	Sweet, bitter, acrid
Sweet Potato	Neutral	Sweet
Taro	Neutral	Acrid
Yamaimo	Neutral	Sweet

Cool foods

Type	Thermal Nature	Flavor
Beer	Cool	Bitter, sweet
White wine	Cool	Sour, sweet
Uron Tea	Cool	Bitter, sweet, astringent
Butter	Cool	Sweet, fatty
Buttermilk	Cool	Sweet
Cottage Cheese	Cool	Sweet, sour
Cream cheese	Cool	Sweet
Sour cream	Cool	Sour, sweet

Type	Thermal Nature	Flavor
Turtle	Cool	Salty
Sea urchins	Cool	Sweet, salty
Soy sauce	Cool	Salty
Avocado	Cool	Sweet
Banana	Cool	Sweet
Blackberry	Cool	Sweet, sour
Blackthorn	Cool	Sour
Blueberry	Cool	Sweet, sour
Cranberry	Cool	Sweet, sour
Currant, red	Cool	Sweet, sour
Gooseberry	Cool	Sweat, sour
Lemon	Cool	Sour, astringent
Mango	Cool	Sweet, sour
Melon	Cool	Sweet, aromatic
Mirabelle	Cool	Sweet, sour
Mulberry	Cool	Sweet, sour
Orange	Cool	Sweet, sour
Passion	Cool	Bitter, bland
Pear	Cool	Sweet, sour
Pomelo	Cool	Sweet, sour
Quince	Cool	Bitter
Star fruit	Cool	Sweet, sour
Strawberry	Cool	Sweet, sour
Tangerine	Cool	Sweet, sour
Barley	Cool	Sweet, salty
Buckwheat	Cool	Sweet
Job's tears	Cool	Sweet, bland
Millet	Cool	Sweet, salty

Type	Thermal Nature	Flavor
Wheat	Cool	Sweet
Wheat bran	Cool	Sweet
Lima bean	Cool	Sweet
Mung bean	Cool	Sweet
Tofu	Cool	Sweet
Duck	Cool	Sweet
Frog	Cool	Sweet
Horse	Cool	Acrid, bitter
Mushroom	Cool	Sweet, bland
Olive Oil	Cool	Sweet, fatty
Wheat vinegar	Cool	Sour
Irish Moss	Cool	Sweet. Salty
Borage	Cool	Bitter, sweet, salty
Chervil	Cool	Bitter, sweet
Lavender	Cool	Bitter, acrid
Marjoram	Cool	Acrid
Mint	Cool	Acrid
Peppermint	Cool	Acrid
Water chestnut	Cool	Sweet, bland
Watercress	Cool	Acrid, bitter
Alfalfa sprouts	Cool	Bitter
Artichoke	Cool	Bitter, sweet
Arugula	Cool	Acrid, bitter
Bok Choy	Cool	Sweet
Burdock root	Cool	Acrid, bitter
Celery	Cool	Sweet, bitter
Chard	Cool	Sweet, bitter
Eggplant	Cool	Sweet

Type	Thermal Nature	Flavor
Endive	Cool	Bitter, sweet
Parsley	Cool	Sweet
Konjac	Cool	Sweet
Lettuce	Cool	Bitter, sweet
Lovage	Cool	Bitter, acrid
Napa cabbage	Cool	Sweet
Radish	Cool	Acrid, sweet
Sauerkraut	Cool	Sour
Sorrel	Cool	Sour
Soybean sprout	Cool	Sweet
Spinach	Cool	Sweet
Tomato	Cool	Sweet, sour
Turnip	Cool	Acrid, bitter
Zucchini	Cool	Sweet, bitter

Cold foods

Type	Thermal Nature	Flavor
Green tea	Cold	Bitter, sweet, astringent
Asari clam	Cold	Sweet, salty
Basket clams	Cold	Sweet, salty
Caviar	Cold	Salty
Crab	Cold	Sweet, salty
Hamaguri	Cold	Salty
Miso	Cold	Salty
Grapefruit	Cold	Sweet, sour
Kiwi	Cold	Sweet, sour

Type	Thermal Nature	Flavor
Persimmon	Cold	Sweet, astringent
Watermelon	Cold	Sweet
Agar (kanten)	Cold	Sweet
Hijiki Seaweed	Cold	Salty
Kelp	Cold	Salty
Nori	Cold	Sweet, salty
Myoga ginger	Cold	Bitter, sweet
Salt	Cold	Salty
Asparagus	Cold	Sweet, bitter
Bamboo Shoots	Cold	Sweet
Bitter melon	Cold	Sweet, bitter
Cucumber	Cold	Sweet, bitter
Rhubarb	Cold	Sour
Rhubarb root	Cold	Bitter

Kampo diagnosis methods

The way you should observe the general and specific appearance of a patient can provide vital information toward revealing the patients specific sho (disease or affliction). Thorough observation, the Kampo practitioner may be able to determine specific sho of the patient, such as whether or not the patient is exhibiting yin or yang sho, or having an indication of Kekkyo-sho (blood deficiency), or Oketsu-sho (blood stasis). The specific characteristics of each sho often manifest in their body shape, posture, and skin complexion.

In both Kampo and traditional Chinese medicine, a close observation of the tongue is an important part of evaluating the health of the patient. The tongue often presents strong visual indicators of a person's overall harmony or disharmony. To perform a tongue diagnosis, the practitioner typically asks the patient to stick out their tongue for observation. The practitioner will then evaluate the size, shape, color, and coating of the tongue. To perform an accurate assessment, it is important for the patient to avoid any activities that may influence the appearance of their tongue prior to the examination, such as consumption of certain artificially-colored foods drinks, or candy. Patients who will be having their tongues inspected are also warned against brushing the surface of their tongue.

While tongue color and coating provide important information, such as signs of blood or Ki (ch'i) vascular, heat, or blood stasis, these observations can be hugely influenced by the lighting in the examination room. Another important part of the tongue evaluation is the observation of sublingual veins, found on the bottom side of the tongue. Patients whose tongues exhibit inadequate shape, length, and or thickness may be indicating signs of blood stasis.

Asking the patient:

The inquiry stage involves asking the patient about his or her medical history, as well as asking if the patient has any current medical complaints or active symptoms.

Modern Kampo practitioners are required to understand and be able to explain the pathophysiology of different diseases in both Western and Eastern terms. Kampo practitioners inquire about patient's illnesses by asking similar questions that Western doctors would ask, including ones regarding previous medical treatments and examinations such as blood tests or X-rays that patients may have had in the past.

In addition to using Western methodology, Kampo practitioners will cover a broad range of other questions, such as asking patients if they have any feelings of warmness or coldness, changes in their appetite or sleep cycles, or difficulty with elimination. In addition, the Kampo practitioner will inquire into the patient's emotional status, their perspiration, their menstruation, all to gain further insight into the patient's health. All of those questions have a specific Eastern diagnostic meanings, and are thus very important.

Hearing:

At this stage of analysis, practitioners will evaluate the tone of voice and the sound the patient makes when they breathe. For example, should the patient have a loud talking voice, that could suggest Jitsu-sho (replete pattern) while patients with soft and quiet voices often indicate the Kikyo-sho (diagnosis of qi vacuity pattern). In some cases, the patient's various odors provide additional clues to help determine diagnosis. A strong odor, for instance, may indicate a heat/excess condition, while a patient with only slight or no odor may indicate a cold/deficiency condition.

The pulse:

It has always amazed me that Western medicine has never caught on to the fact about taking a pulse in various parts of the body can lead to uncovering health issues and no equipment is needed.

The classic "six areas to take a pulse".
With regard to pulse diagnosis, Western doctors are known to conduct this procedure, but only in a limited fashion. They usually only evaluate the rate of a patient's pulse, using the procedure to count beats per minute, for instance. In contrast, Oriental medicine practitioners evaluate patient's pulse in far more detail, focusing on the pulse's quality and if it exhibits different characteristics:

Pulse characteristics may indicate conditions related to heat or cold, acute or chronic states, vacuity or repletion states, and other constitutional patterns and difficulties. A method of pulse diagnosis in "six positions" may also be used to determine a potential organ or meridian imbalance. However, Oriental pulse diagnosis has been criticized as highly subjective means of examination. It is considered an art more than it is a science. In order to obtain more accurate and reliable pulse information from patients, practitioners need to be fully aware of the fact that cardiovascular functions are instantly and profoundly affected by various environmental factors and common activities such as posture, respiration, and mental alertness etc. Accordingly, those factors and activities can influence almost all basic categories of classical pulse including Speed, Strength, Size, Tension, and Flow. It is very important to carefully consider and control various influential factors while assessing the patient. Only then, the pulse diagnosis, when conducted skillfully, can provide useful and vital information about patient's illness or constitution.

Examination of the abdominal area:

The abdominal diagnosis, a practice known as Fukushin is unique to the Kampo School. This practice is not included in modern iterations of traditional Chinese medicine. Fukushin is considered one of the most vital parts of the Kampo diagnosis procedure. It has been found to have a relatively higher intra- and inter-examiner correlation than what was found through studies of pulse analysis.

Fukushin is different compared to other abdominal palpation commonly performed by Western physicians, at least in terms of its intent and procedure. In Western medicine, the main purpose of palpation is to attempt to feel a patient's organs through their body surface. In this scenario, a patient's knee is bended to minimize the interference of their abdominal muscles.

In Kampo, abdominal diagnosis is usually conducted while patient's leg is fully extended, being that its primary purpose is to evaluate the responses reflected by the surface of the patient's body.

The appearance of bloating, should be noted as a digestive problem and should be taken seriously. This should allow you to ask the patient about the diet they currently follow.

Kampo herbs

The herbs used in kampo, are not limited to all the ones I have listed. They can amount to thousands of different herbal combinations and also single herbs combined with certain foods may provide relief to what ails you.

Something to keep in mind if you are used to the Western medicine prescription "drugs". Kampo herbs and formulas, are subtle. They act in a slower (yet safer) way and few (if any side effects). This can take a matter of hours, days, weeks and even months to bring you back to health. Depending on your condition and how long you have been afflicted with it.

Remember if it took time to get into your present state of un-health(i.e. fat over-weight, lack of energy, etc.). It will take time to get back into a good to excellent state of health.

Too many people in this society want the instant 'microwave' treatment, and these come with harsh side effects and often lead to other health problems. I have seen this in athletes who want to be faster, bigger in muscle size, and stronger, use chemical enhancements. Instead of training and eating correctly for a committed span of ten years or more. They end up aged prematurely and then have a host of side effects and other health issues to deal with the rest of their lives, for a short lived athletic career.

I can only hope that the youth will look into the long term effects of what they do to themselves now will affect them after the age of thirty. To which I have noted a surprising amount of teenagers today do not even think they will be alive then? This pessimistic attitude must be changed by the parents, teachers, and mentors of our world, to a optimistic one.

All herbs should be cycled in an on and off basis of taking them. This includes favorites like; ginseng root, Ho Shou wu (Fo-Ti), etc. The reason for doing this is because after approximately six to eight weeks your cell receptor sites in your body, will get used to the herb(s) being used.

In order for you to get the same effect from the herb(s) you would need to increase the dosage this is what you do not want to do. It is far better to take a break for six to eight weeks. Abstaining from the herb(s) being used will clear your cells receptor sites (make fresh) and you can resume the same dosage as before for another six to eight weeks.

The other treatment yo may also wish to do is use another herb(s) during your abstaining period from six to eight weeks. This is another excellent method for continued health and treatment of any "sho" or desired health benefit you want (i.e. extra libido for a honeymoon period, or needing extra stamina). This is permitted as long as you do not become addicted to the herb(s) being used or combination thereof.

It has been my experience to always maintain a balance in all aspects of life. We all have certain circumstances that will not allow this to happen. But these are always short lived and you can look back on your life and see you were focused too intensely on the problem at hand to note that it would not be that way forever.

List of main Kampo herbs

Japanese   Chinese   English
gaiyo......ai ye......wormwood leaf, mugwort leaf
(Artemisiae Capillari Flos).

hazu.......ba dou.....croton seed
(Crotonis Fructus).

byakug.....bai he.....tiger lily bulb
(Lilii Bulbus).
byakushi...bai zhi....angelica root
(Angelicae dahuricae Radix).

byakujutst.bai zhu....white atractylodes rhizome
(Atractylodis macrocephalae).

hanmyo.....ban mao....mylabris,
(cantharides   Mylabris).

hange......ban xia....pinellia rhizome
(Pinelliae Rhizoma).

baimo......bei mu.....fritillaria bulb
(Fritillariae Bulbus).

hamabofu...bei sha shen..glehnia rhizome
(Glehniae Radix Cum Rhizoma).

Japanese   Chinese   English

binroji....bing lang...betel nut/areca nut (Arecae Semen).

hakka......bo he.......wild mint herb (Menthae haplocalycis Herba).

sojutsu....cangzhu.....atractylodes rhizome (Atractylodis Lanceae Rhizoma).

sokuhakuyo.ce bai ye..Oriental arborvitae leafy twig   (Platycladi Cacumen).

chayo......cha ye.....tea leaf (Camelliae Folium).

saiko......chai hu....bupleurum root (Bupleuri Radix).

senso......chan su....toad venom (Bufonis Venenum).

zentai.....chan tui...cicada molting (Cicadae Periostracum).

shazenshi..che qian zi..Chinese plantain seed (Plantaginis Semen).

Japanese   Chinese   English

chinpi.....chen pi....aged mikan orange peel (Citri reticulatae Pericarpium).

jinko......chen xiang..aquilaria wood, aloeswood (Aquilariae Lignum resinatum).

senkotsu...chuan gu...Japanese water lily rhizome (Nupharis Rhizoma).

senkyu.....chuan xiong...cnidium root (Chuanxiong Rhizoma).

daifukuhi..da fu pi.....areca husk, areca peel (Arecae Pericarpium).

daio.......da huang.....turkey rhubarb rhizome

(Rhei Rhizoma).

taiso......da zao.....jujube fruit, Chinese date (Jujubae Fructus).

taishaseke.dai zhe shi....hematite (Haematitum).

takuchikuyo.dan zhu ye...lophatherum stem and leaves (Lophatheri Herba).

Japanese   Chinese   English

toki.......dang gui..Chinese angelica root (Angelicae sinensis Radix).

jikoppi....di gu pi..wolfberry tree bark (Lycii Cortex).

jio........di huang..rehmannia root, Chinese foxglove root (Rehmanniae Radix).

chotoko....diao gou teng...gambier extract (Uncariae Uncis Cum Ramulus).

choko......ding xiang....clove (Caryophylli Flos).

choji......ding zi....clove flower (Caryophylli Flos).

tochukaso..dong chong xia cao..cordyceps, Chinese caterpillar fungus   (Cordyceps).

togashi....dong gua zi...winter melon seed (Benincasae Semen).

tochu......du zhong...eucommia bark (Eucommiae Cortex).

Japanese   Chinese   English

akyo.......e jiao....collagen
(Asini Corii Colla).

bofu.......fang feng....saposhnikovia root
(Saposhnikoviae Radix).

bukuryo....fu ling.....tuckahoe mushroom
(Poria).

bu shi.....fu zi...Carmichael's monkshood rhizome
(Aconiti Rhizoma).

kanzo......gan cao....Chinese liquorice root
   (Glycyrrhizae Radix).

kankyo.....gan jiang...dried ginger rhizome
   (Zingiberis Siccatum Rhizoma).

kakkon.....ge gen...kudzu root
(Puerariae Radix).

gokai......ge jie...gecko
(Gecko).

kukoshi....gou qi zi...wolfberry tree fruit
   (Lycii Fructus).

Japanese   Chinese   English

karokon....gua lou gen...trichosanthes root
(Trichosanthis Radix).

karonin....gua lou ren...trichosanthes seed
(Trichosantis Semen).

keihi......gui pi...Chinese cinnamon bark
(Cinnamomi Cortex).

keishi.....gui zhi....cinnamon twig
(Cinnamomi Ramulus).

kaikujin...hai gou shen...male seal sexual organs
(Callorhini Testes et Penis).

kashu......he shou wu (Fo-Ti)...Chinese knotweed
(Polygoni Multiflori Radix).

kashi......he zi   chebule,myrobalan-fruit,
terminalia, chebgium
(Chebulae Fructus).

koka.......hong hua....safflower flower
(Carthami Flos).

koboku.....hou po...magnolia bark
(Magnoliae officinalis Cortex).

Japanese   Chinese   English

goma.......hu ma...sesame seed
(Sesami Semen).

kasseki....hua shi...talcum powder
(Talcum Crystallinum).

obaku......huang bai...cork-tree bark
(Phellodendri Cortex).

osei.......huang jing...polygonatum rhizome,
Siberian Solomon's seal   (Polygonati Rhizoma).

oren.......huang lian...goldenthread rhizome
(Coptidis Rhizoma).

ogi........huang qi...astragalus root
(Astragali Radix).

ogon.......huang qin...skullcap root
(Scutellariae Radix).

uikyo......hui xiang...fennel fruit
(Foeniculi Fructus).

kakko......huo xiang...pogostemon
(Pogostemonis, Agstaches Herba).

Japanese   Chinese   English
shitsurishi.ji li zi caltrop fruit, puncture vine fruit, tribulus
(Tribuli Fructus).

koi........jiao yi...ground sugar
(Saccharum Granorum).

kikyo.......jie geng...Chinese bellflower root, balloon flower root
(Platycodi Radix).

kinginka....jin yin hua...honeysuckle flower, lonicera   (Lonicerae Flos).

keigai......jing jie...schizonepeta spikes
(Schizonepetae Herba).

koubei......jing mi...rice seed
(Oryzae Semen).

kikuka......ju hua...chrysanthemum flower
(Chrysanthemi Flos).

ketsumeishi.jue ming zi...cassia seed   (Cassiae Semen).

kujin.......ku shen...sophora root
(Sophorae flavescentis Radix).

Japanese   Chinese   English

kantoka....kuan dong hua...coltsfoot
(Farfarare Flos).

rengyo.....lian qao...forsythia fruit
(Forsythiae Fructus).

rensenso...lian qian cao...glechoma, longtube ground ivy   (Glechomae Herba).

renniku....lian rou...sacred lotus seed
(Nelumbis Semen).

renshi.....lian zi...lotus seed
(Nelumbinis Semen).

ryokyo.....liang jiang...lesser galangal rhizome
(Alpiniae Officinari Rhizoma).

reiyokaku..ling yang cao...antelope horn
(Saigae tataricae Cornu).

ryutan.....long dan cao...Chinese gentian root
(Gentianae Scabrae Radix).

ryukotsu...long gu...dragon bone, fossilized vertebrae and bones
(Fossilia Ossis Mastodi).

Japanese   Chinese   English

ryuganniku.long yan rou...longan fruit flesh
(Longan Arillus).

rokujo.....lu rong...deer velvet
(Cervi Cornu pantotrichum).

mao........ma huang...ephedra herb
(Ephedrae Herba).

bakuga.....ma ya...Barley sprouts, malt Hordei
(Fructus Germinatus).

mashinin...ma zi ren...hemp fruit
(Cannabis Fructus).

bakumondo..mai men dong...mondo grass rhizome, ophiopogon tuber
(Ophiopogonis Radix).

mankeishi..man jing zi...vitex fruit
(Viticis Fructus).

bosho......mang xiao...sodium sulfate
(Natrii Sulfus).

botanpi....mu dan pi...tree peony bark
(Paeoniae Moutan Cortex).

Japanese   Chinese   English
mokuboi....mu fang ji.Cocculi root
(Cocculi Radix).

mokka......mu gua chaenomeles...fruit Chinese quince fruit
(Chaenomelis Fructus).

borei......mu li   pacific oyster shell
(Ostreae Concha).

mokutsu....mu tong   chocolate vine stem
(Akebiae Caulis).

mokko......mu xiang   saw-wort root, snow lotus root
(Aucklandiae Radix).

goboshi....niu bang zi   greater burdock fruit
(Arcti Fructus).

goshitsu...niu xi achyranthis root
(Achyranthis bidentatae Radix).

goo........niu huang   cattle gallstone
(Bovis Calculus).

biwayo.....pi pa ye   loquat leaf
(Eriobotryae Folium).

Japanese   Chinese   English

hokoei.....pu gong ying   dandelion, taraxacum
(Taraxaci Herba).

kyokatsu...qiang huo   notopterygium rhizome
(Notopterygii Rhizoma seu Radix).

jingyo.....qin jiao   large   gentian root,
gentiana macrophylla root
(Gentianae macrophyllae Radix).

boi........qing feng teng   Sesami Semen
(Sinomeni Caulis et Rhizoma).

zenko......quan hu   persicae semen
(Peucedani Radix).

nindo......ren dong teng Japanese honeysuckle stem   (Lonicerae Folium Cum Caulis).

ninjin.....ren shen   ginseng root
(Ginseng Radix).

nikujuyo...rou cong rong   cistanche, broomrape
(Cistanche Herba).

sohakuhi...sang bai pi   mulberry root bark
(Mori Cortex).

Japanese   Chinese   English

soyo.......sang ye   white mulberry leaf
(Mori Folium).

shukusha...sha ren   black cardamom seed
(Amomi Semen).

sanyaku....shan yao   Chinese yam rhizome
(Dioscoreae Rhizoma).

sanzashi...shan zha   Japanese hawthorn fruit
(Crataegi Fructus).

sanshishi..shan zhi zi   gardenia fruit
(Gardeniae Fructus).

sanshuyu...shan zhu yu   Japanese cornel fruit
(Corni Fructus).

shakuyaku..shao yao   Chinese peony root
(Paeoniae Radix).

jashoshi...she chuang zi   cnidium seed
(Cinidii Fructus).

jako.......she xiang   musk-deer
(Moschus).

Japanese   Chinese   English

shokyo.....sheng jiang   fresh ginger rhizome
    (Zingiberis Rhizoma).

shoma......sheng ma   cemicifuga,bugbane rhizome,
black cohosh rhizome   (Cimicifugae Rhizoma).

sekko......shi gao   gypsum mineral
(Gypsum fibrosum).

sekkoku....shi hu   dendrobium
(Dendrobii Herba).

sekketsumei.shi jue ming   abalone shell
(Halitotidis Concha).

shikunshi..shi jun zi   rangoon creeper fruit
with seeds, quisqualis   (Quisqualis Fructus).

soboku.....su mu   sappan wood shavings
(Sappan Lignum).

sansonin...suan zao ren   sour jujube seed
(Zizyphi Spinosae Semen).

tonin......tao ren   peach kernel
(Persicae Semen).

Japanese   Chinese   English

tenma......tian ma   gastrodia rhizome
(Gastrodiae Rhizoma).

tenmondo...tian men dong asparagus root
(Asparagi Radix).

tennansho..tian nan xing arisaema rhizome
(Arisaematis Rhizoma).

shachu.....tu bie chong   ground beetle, wingless cockroach   (Eupolyphaga).

dokkatsu...tu dang gui   Japanese spikenard rhizome   (Araliae pubescentis Radix, Cordatae Rhizoma).

dobukuryo...tu fu ling   smooth greenbrier rhizome, smilax
(Smilacis glabrae Rhizoma).

gomishi....we wei zi schisandra fruit
(Schisandrae Fructus).

ireisen....wei ling xian clematis root
(Clematidis Radix).

gobaishi...wu bei zi   gallnut of Chinese sumac

Japanese   Chinese   English

gokahi.....wu jia pi   acanthopanax root bark, eleutherococus root bark (Acanthopanacis Cortex).

uyaku......wu yao   spicebush root, benjamin bush root   (Linderae Radix).

goshuyu....wu zhu yu   evodia fruit (Evodiae Fructus).

saikaku....xi jiao   rhinoceros horn (Rhinocerotis Cornu).

saishin....xi xin   asarum, Chinese wild ginger (Asari Radix et Rhizoma).

kagoso.....xia ku cao   prunella, selfheal spike (Prunellae Spica).

kobushi....xiang fu zi   nut-grass rhizome (Cyperi Rhizoma).

bokusoku...xiang shi   sawtooth oak bark (Quercus Cortex).

shoubaku...xiao mai   wheat seed

Japanese   Chinese   English

shini......xin yi willow-leafed magnolia flower
(Magnoliae Flos).

kyonin.....xing ren   apricot kernel
(Armeniacae Semen).

yutan......xion dan   bear gallbladder
(Vesica Fellea Ursi).

senpukuka..xuan fu hua   inula flower   inulae
(Flos).

engosaku...yan hu suo   corydalis rhizome
(Corydalis Rhizoma).

yakumoso...yi mu cao Chinese motherwort herb
(Leonuri Herba).

yokuinin...yi yi ren job's tears seed
(Coicis Semen).

inchinko...yin chen hao   capillary wormwood
(Artemisia Capillaris Thunb).

inyokaku...yin yang huo   epimedium
(Epimedii Herba).

Japanese   Chinese   English

ukon.......yu jin curcuma tuber (Curcumae Radix).

juyaku.....yu xing cao   houttuynia (Houttuyniae Herba).

onji.......yuan zhi   milkwort root, snakeroot (Polygalae Radix).

takusha....ze xie water plantain rhizome (Alismatis Rhizoma).

shakanzo...zhi gan cao   Chinese liquorice root (Glycyrrhizae Radix preparata).

kikoku.....zhi ke bitter orange (Auranti Fructus).

chimo......zhi mu anemarrhena rhizome (Anemarrhenae Rhizoma).

kijitsu....zhi shi   unripe bitter orange (Auranti Fructus immaturus).

chikusetsuninjin...zhu jie ren shen Japanese ginseng root   (Panacis Japonicus).

Japanese   Chinese   English

chorei...zhu ling   polyporus mushroom (Polyporus).

chikujo...zhu ru   bamboo shavings (Bambusae Caulis, Phyllostachysis Caulis).

shusha...zhu sha   cinnabar (Cinnabaris).

shikon...zi gen   lithospermum root (Lithospermi Radix).

shisoyo...zi su ye   perilla leaf (Perillae Folium).

* Note on Ho Shou wu (Fo-Ti), is the main herb that is much safer than ginseng. That helps tone up all the human body's glands and aides in keeping the vascular linings of both arteries and veins elastic and relatively plaque free!
  Much more research should be done on this amazing herb and its properties. It has also been demonstrated to keep hair from turning gray, reducing inflamation, keeping your healthy youth like energy well into what is considered "old age".

Anti-aging herbs:

Kava Kava is used to aid anxiety. It will help you to relax and sleep well.

Plum Flower products are used to treat people who suffer with various illnesses, including migraines, hypertension, cancers, heart disease, gastro intestine problems, and common headaches.

Gui Pi Wan supplements are great for workaholic. This herb works to nourish the mind.

Eleuthero will support the system by providing you with improved blood circulation.

Ginkgo Biloba is a great herb that increases blood circulation and it will help the lungs function properly, while distributing or promoting oxygen flow, which will in turn produces freedom of blood flowing to the brain. For those suffering with memory loss or forgetfulness it support healthy brain functions. It is designed to enhance mental alertness.

Alfalfa (Medicago sativa) contains tremendous amount of concentrations of chlorophyll. This is the pigment that is responsible for the fresh green look found in the plants. Chlorophyll will aid in ridding the body of old depleted cells replacing them with brand new ones that are healthy to the body.

Aloe Vera is an ingredient in many beauty products, especially lotion and shampoos and also other skin care products. Its usefulness as an herbal medicine is numerous but it is a good anti aging herb that can also retards aging. Some individuals including myself, use the gel as a face mask to prevent wrinkles and acne. This plant possesses elements that will soothe and smooth the skin and it is also a very good laxative herb.

Tea tree oil is deemed an excellent natural herbal antiseptic and is also an ingredient in many products related to beauty care. It is very good to treat acne as well as skin conditions.

Anti-anxiety herbs:

Anxiety can be erased naturally with anxiety herbs. People try various methods to combat anxiety, but the following medicinal herbs for anxiety are very beneficial in treating anxiety.

Ginseng: It can help a person who is suffering from stress and anxiety by reducing these ailments. This is an alternative to the popular anti-depressant medications that may not be effective. It is also said that one of the best hair loss treatment is ginseng.

Valerian: This is one of the anxiety herbs that is used against sleeping disorders, restlessness and anxiety. Its therapeutic effects are positive and will especially benefits those who suffer insomnia.

Catnip: Herbal tea are is a good thing when it comes to fighting insomnia and catnip tea is one of them. It is very soothing and can induce sleep and it will aid in alleviating headaches.

Damiana: This is used to treat depression and anxiety which affect thousands of people worldwide.

Chamomile: Chamomile is a tonic and a stimulant herb which is a relaxant for stress and anxiety. It is one of the top ten herbs for relaxation and calm. Drinking the chamomile herbal tea can soothe the nerves and gives anyone a good night's sleep.

Bugleweed: This is a sedative herb and will calm the mind.

St. John's Wort: This is yet another potent herb that is used for hysteria and nervousness. It is also seen as a very prominent and primary medicinal herb to aid in stressful conditions.

Lemon balm: This medicinal herb is used to reduce stress and compounds are found in it which are responsible for calming as well as sedative effect when it is consumed.

kava kava: Kava kava gives the feeling of mental clarity and it is a very good and natural remedy to aid in stress and anxiety. It can also be found in some breast enhancement creams.

Ashwagandha: Effective in decreasing stress and increasing mental activity.

Passionflower: is also an excellent herb to treat this ailment. It can encourage relation and calmness in a person and it can also treat sleeping disorders.

Herbal anxiety treatments: Can improve your life and free you from the grip that anxiety has over your life. Anxiety can be too painful for many to endure. Learn natural ways to treat and cure anxiety.
Anxiety herbs are really the answer to stress and nervous conditions and can give medicinal benefits to thousands of people who suffer from these conditions every day.

Anti-high blood pressure herbs:

Blood pressure herbs are considered to be most effective in treating high blood pressure (hypertension) or low blood pressure (hypotension).
Millions of people all over the world are being treated for high blood pressure. Every year many of these people die as a result of this condition. Some occur from a blood clot that travels to the brain which is referred to as a stroke caused by high blood pressure.

There are those who have survived this ordeal but are unable to take care of themselves because the stroke caused them to be disabled.

High blood pressure or hypertension is defined as having blood pressure equal to or higher than 160 systolic (the top number) over 95 diastolic (the bottom number). Between 140 and 159 systolic over 90 to 94 diastolic is also considered high or borderline, however below these numbers are considered to be normal.

There are natural ways to lower blood pressure which include exercise and diet but herbal medicine in the form of medicinal herbs, is perhaps the most potent natural cure for high blood pressure.

The blood pressure herbs to lower blood pressure are garlic, black cohosh, blue cohosh, hyssop, wild black cherry bark, valerian, vervain, sanicle, boneset, skullcap, goldenseal, Indian spikenard and myrrh.

Garlic tablets and garlic water will help to regulate blood pressure. It is written that dried watermelon seed made into a tea will bring down high blood pressure.

The avocado leaves medicinal herbs are also very effective medicinal benefits in lowering high blood pressure.

Low blood pressure herbs

Low Blood Pressure (Hypotension)

Most people's attention is centered on High blood Pressure, but low blood pressure is just as dangerous. For many years, I troubled with low blood pressure, so I am talking from experience. Thank God, my blood pressure in now normal.

Blood pressure is the force of blood pushing against the walls of the arteries as the heart pumps out blood.

If it is lower than normal then it is called low blood pressure or hypotension. If it is higher than normal then it is called high blood pressure or hypertension.

Pressure below 110/70mmHg is considered low. It makes you feel weak, tired, and dizzy. If your blood pressure remains too low for extended periods, it can cause damage to the liver, heart, and other organs. It can even cause death.

Chinese herbal medicine for high blood pressure

Chinese healing herbs may also be included in blood pressure herbs because they are also very effective for both conditions.

It is said in Chinese medicine that symptoms related to high blood pressure (hypertension) are mostly connected to a pattern that is referred to as Liver Heat or Yang Rising. Some of these symptoms are pressure behind the eyes, headaches as well as dizziness.

Therefore to manage high blood pressure naturally, Chinese herbal medicine as well as acupuncture may be utilized. In this Chinese herbal medicine, there are anti-hypertensive herbs or high blood pressure herbs that may be proven quite effective. There are also medicinal herbs that may be used to manage high cholesterol and at the same time boost the functions of cardiovascular conditions.

Acupuncture can bring about a very calming and relaxed effect which can be very helpful in hypertension and stressful conditions. These are commonly utilized in treating the patterns that related to hypertension (high blood pressure.) A primary medicinal herb that is used for patterns and symptoms for high blood pressure is **gastrodia rhizome** or **Tian Ma**, which may be termed as high blood pressure herb.

Scientific studies in China has discovered Tian Ma can be very useful to treat the symptoms of high blood pressure such as tinnitus, dizziness, headaches, numbness of limbs of the body as well as pain and aches behind the eyes. Tian Ma or gastrodia rhizome possesses calming and sedative effects and has been proven to be useful in the treatment of essential hypertension as well as renal hypertension.

Other blood pressure treatment

Other methods to help treat high blood pressure is to:
• Steam the **breadfruit blossom** and drink the water. Also a tea of the breadfruit leaves is very effective.
• Drink **chocho** juice.
• Put a spoonful of **cream of tarter** in some water and drink it.
•Drinking **garlic water** may help to reduce high blood pressure which is also referred to as hypertension.

Apple cider vinegar can be included in blood pressure herbs. It is very good to treat low blood pressure. Also beet root juice is most effective.

Remember at all times to contact your doctor if you think you are suffering from high or low blood pressure because these two conditions can be very fatal. Also, tell your doctor about the blood pressure herbs that you are using for medicinal benefits.

Diabetes herbs that may help:

The following herbs are listed together and may help in the treatment of diabetes or lessen the need for diabetic drugs.

Saw palmetto, Eucalyptus leaf, Dandelion root, Uva urs, Buchu, Blueberry leaf, Golden seal, Gymnema Sylvestre, Blue cohosh, Raspberry leaf, Periwinkle, and Garlic.

Herbs for hayfever relief:

Medicinal herbs for hay fever are goldenseal, ragweed (some people are allergic to this herb), golden rod, skunk cabbage, bayberry bark as well as calamus root, butterbur (this will help with breathing), eyebright, nettle leaf and ephedra.

A teaspoonful each of goldenseal and borax combined with one pint of boiling water should be good. Shake this combination well and allow to stand for two hours, while shaking it periodically. After the two hours pour some of it in the hand and inhale with one nostril at a time. This process, while doing it for a number of times, will eventually clean the nose and bring healing to the membranes.

A mixture of one teaspoonful each of the calamus root, goldenrod, ragweed and the skunk cabbage is a good combination. Then one teaspoonful of this mixture may be placed in a glass of warm water and consumed one hour before meal and or upon retiring to bed.

A continuous drinking of herbal drinks as well as herbal teas can be quite effective in treating hay fever.

Steep one tablespoon full of ephedra may be placed in one pint of boiling water for one and a half hour. Then strain this mixture through a piece of cloth and sniff it through the nostrils. This may be done three to four times daily until relief is felt.

Apart from hay fever herbs, it is also said that sufferers may used warm salt water to gargle the throat.

Herbs for prostate relief:

Medicinal herbs such as, **parsley, uva ursi, ginger, juniper berry, gravel root, echinacea, red clover, yucca, goldenseal, couch grass, licorice root, kelp, pumpkin seeds, joe-pye weed root, corn silk, saw palmetto berries, white pond lily, buchu, alfalfa and garlic** are used to treat these diseases.

Treatment can include surgery, radiation and hormones all of which have long-term effects on men's quality of life when it comes to sexual function. Medicinal herbs are milder and safer to use.

Other herbal treatment for this dreaded disease is by making a poultice from one of the prostate herbs which is slippery elm and then place it between the legs, near to the crotch to ease pain.

Make a tea of equal parts of **buchu** and **uva ursi** of a teaspoonful, add to a cup of boiling water then, allow to simmer then drink one to four cups per day.

Prostate conditions may also be aided by the unique **Aloe Vera** plant which may also give you double protection against prostate conditions, other diseases, germ and the freedom to live your life.

Lycopene, which is a very potent antioxidant is found in tomato-based meals. It is good for the prostate and therefore these foods are popularly consumed by men because according to scientific researches, they are rich in lycopene and this antioxidant will aid in combating and preventing cancerous cells. Lycopene is also seen as a tumor reducer.

For men who are 40 years and older, it is suggested that you do a yearly rectal examination and with the aid of prostate herbs along with approval of your doctor, you may just decrease the threat of prostate conditions.

Increase testosterone in males:

Damiana: This medicinal plant is used to treat sterility, impotence, diabetes, asthma, bladder infections and respiratory problems. Therefore instead of using chemical medication to cure impotence and sterility, the natural alternative is the use of this plant

Sarsaparilla: In a research done on the root in 1993 at the Pennsylvania State University, the root was found to contain male and female hormones and it is used to treat sterility as well impotence in men.

Gotu kola: It is said that this herb or its tea will increase the vitality of an 80 year old person to that of a forty year old person. It has an energizing effect on the brain cells and can preserve it indefinitely. It is also used to treat sterility as well impotence in men.

Ginseng: Ginseng medicinal herb is an effective remedy for sexual dysfunction in men. Small pieces of the fresh raw root may be eaten daily to aid this problem.

Saw palmetto: This herb boosts the immune system and fights against both male and female infertility as well as it is an effective remedy for sexual dysfunction in men.

Fresh parsley: The raw fresh parsley is a part of herbal impotence remedy and it is also effective to treat this problem.

Pumpkin seeds: Eating a few teaspoonfuls of these seeds prove beneficial.

Tong Kat Ali: Also known as "Long fellow Jack" will increase your libido as well as the free testosterone in your blood stream. This herb can b taken with or without food and has no side effects with a dosage as low as 500 milligrams one can feel the effects in a matter of hours.

Maca root: Is another herb that may increase free testosterone in the blood stream. However this is not reported in all case as with the Tong Kat Ali herb.

Herbal teas such as **fenugreek, strong back, sarsaparilla root, gotu kola, ginseng, joe-pye weed (gravel root), Irish moss as well as corn silk** are also useful and beneficial in regards to herbal testosterone increase.

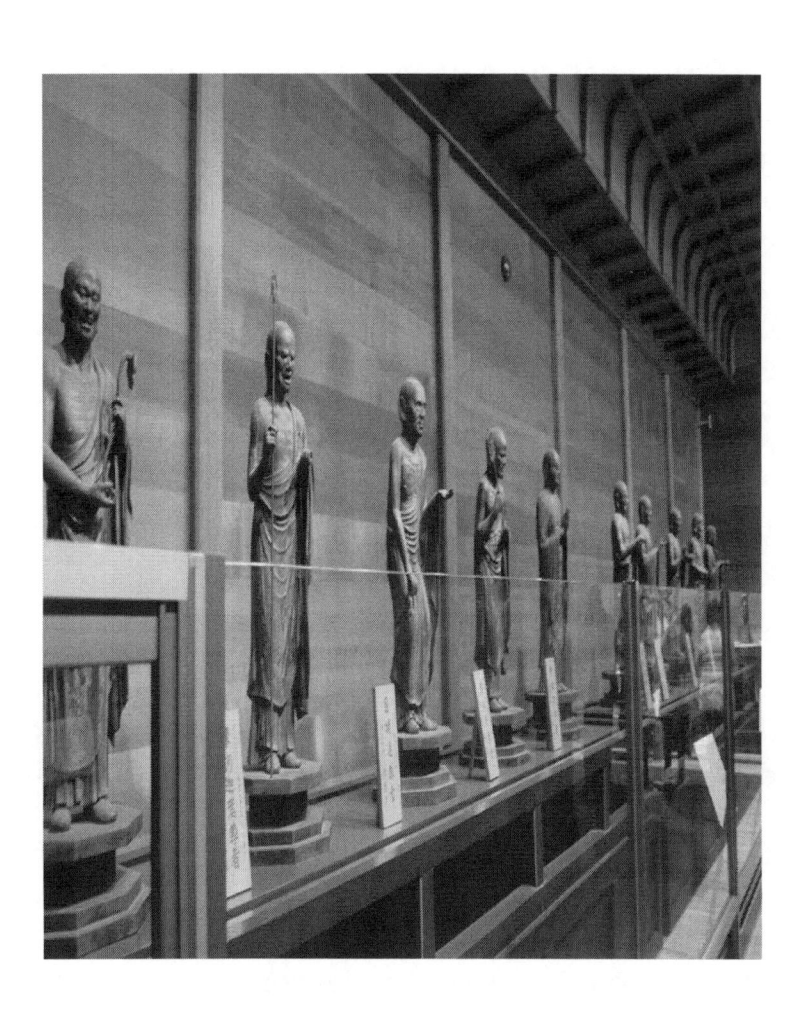

Kampo lifestyle

The lifestyle you follow will directly affect your health and well-being. Eating and drinking correctly will help enormously, but this is only part of your all around health especially when you get older (past middle age).

What you still need is a good amount of regular exercise on a daily (or at least every other day). Some type of exercise you like/love to do and know you will not stop doing even in your advanced years. This can be anything that gets your blood circulating (more than at rest or sitting/lying position) and increases your respiration rate (breathing more and deeper than you would at rest).

The next main component is your will power and being able to exercise that will go a long way to keeping your health in check and desire more out of life. If you have no desire my friend to live-It will not matter. Your health will follow your minds direction, and your will fall into ill health/depression and die.

However, if you do have a desire and lust for life, coupled with a purpose. Then nothing can keep you from obtaining that which you want to do and your health will always be robust.

As you can see by the world ranking of life expectancy. Japan is number one in the world!

No other country is this high despite the high industry, and ultra fast pace way of life.

Region Rank Life expectancy comparison:
1. Japan- Age 82.70

2. Singapore- Age 82.35

3. South Korea- Age 80.72

4. Brunei- Age 77.36

5. Maldives- Age 76.59

6. China- Age 75.56

7. Viet Nam- Age 75.19

8. Sri Lanka- Age 74.56

9. Thailand- Age 74.01

10. Malaysia- Age 73.94

11. Georgia- Age 72.09

12. Azerbaijan- Age 71.41

13. Armenia- Age 71.27

14. Bangladesh- Age 69.52

15. Indonesia- Age 69.47

16. Philippines- Age 69.40

17. Russia- Age 68.85

These are just the average ages. Japan on a regular basis has out ranked all world countries for decades. An interesting note; The Japanese that migrate to America's (both North and South) have not had the continued longevity after the first generation. The second and third generation Japanese American's adapted to the diet and lifestyle the majority of Americans enjoy? With the same unhealthy effects occurring to them;

i.e. high blood pressure, heart attacks, and stroke.

The Western fast food craze has invaded Japan as well and consequently, had a negative impact on the youth especially of Japan. The older and wiser natives of Japan for the most part do not embrace the American fast foods and diet.

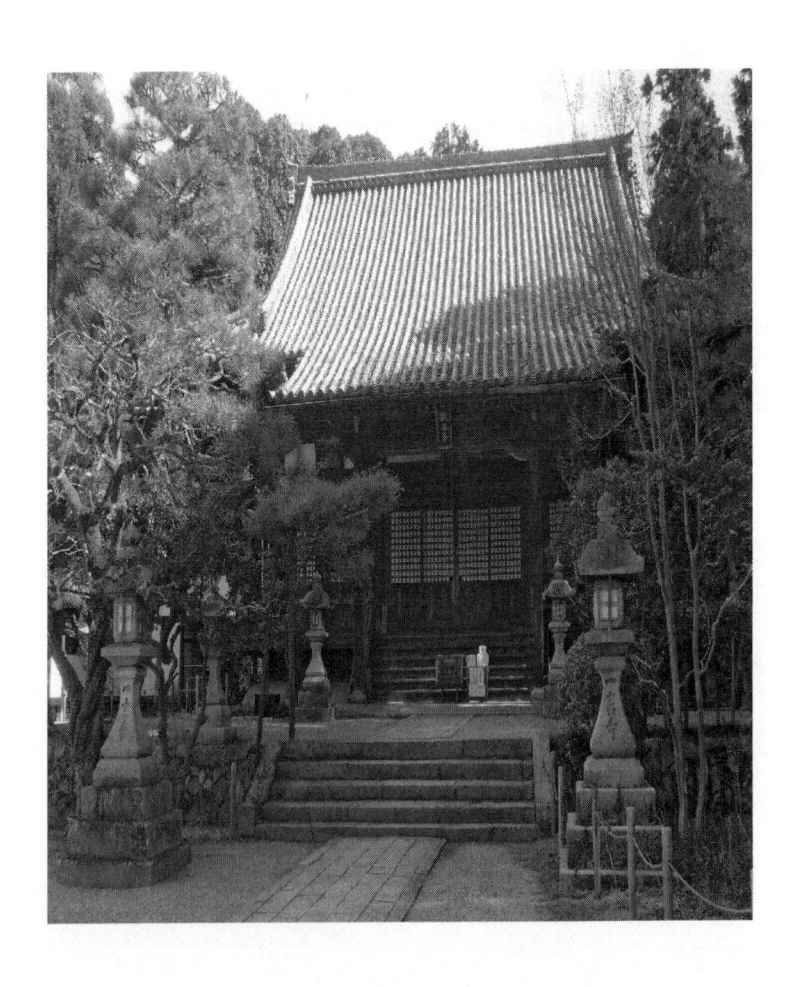

Deer antler-Secret formula used for: Blood, bone, and joint health

Deer antler is a common ingredient in traditional Chinese medicine. It may be surprising, especially to the practitioner of Chinese medicine, to learn that New Zealand is the world's largest producer of deer antler, followed closely by Australia and Canada (both increasing rapidly), and that Korea is probably the world's largest user of antlers, with an apparently insatiable appetite for antlers of all species. China is also a major producer and consumer of deer antler products and appears to have the longest history of medicinal use of deer antler as well as production via deer farming.

The story of deer antler can be traced back to the first Chinese Materia Medica, Shennong Bencao Jing (ca. 100 A.D.), where it is described briefly (1). There is also reference to earlier use of deer antler in an archeological find (a set of silk scrolls named Wushier Bingfang, from a tomb dated 168 B.C.). However, use of antler appears to have been infrequent until the animals were raised on "deer farms" starting in the mid-16th Century in China (Ming Dynasty period). This is a time when several other cultivation and animal husbandry projects were established in support of medicine. Soon after, Wu Kun included a formula in his book Yi Fang Kao (Study of Prescriptions, 1584) that has inspired much work with the combination of deer antler and tortoise shell, two bone-like materials rich in gelatins. His formula is Gui Lu Erxian Jiao (gui = tortoise, lu = deer, erxian = two immortals; jiao = gelatin). The formula is made as a firm gelatin, using the following recipe (proportioned to the amount being made):

Deer antler (lujiao) 5,000 g
Tortoise plastron (guiban) 2,000 g
Lycium fruit (goujizi) 1,500 g
Ginseng (renshen) 500 g

This formula is said to replenish yin and essence, tonify Ki,Ch'i, or qi, and strengthen yang. It is used for deficiency of kidney yin and yang, deficiency of blood and essence in the penetrating and conception vessels, with symptoms of weakness of the lower back and legs, impotence, blurred vision, etc. (2). The penetrating vessel, (chongmai), one of the extra meridians, is referred to as the "sea of blood."

The conception vessel (renmai), while sometimes associated with reproduction, is related to generation more broadly, including generation of blood. Tortoise shell and deer antler are said to nourish the marrow.

More importantly for the future of Chinese herb prescribing with deer antler, Zhang Jingyue described two important tonic formulas in pill form (presented in the book Jingyue Quanshu, 1624), one to emphasize tonification of kidney yang (said to nourish the right kidney), called Yougui Wan, and one to emphasize nourishing kidney yin (said to nourish the left kidney), called Zuogui Wan. Though prepared originally as pills (= wan), they were later commonly used as decoctions for replenishing the kidney (you = right; zuo = left; gui = replenish).

Yougui Wan   Zuogui Wan
Rehmannia (shudi)
Dioscorea (shanyao)
Cornus (shanzhuyu)
Lycium (goujizi)
Cuscuta (tusizi)
Deer antler gelatin (lujiaojiao)
Tang-kuei (danggui)

Eucommia (duzhong)
Cinnamon bark (rougui)
Aconite (fuzi)   Rehmannia (shudi)
Dioscorea (shanyao)
Cornus (shanzhuyu)
Lycium (goujizi)
Cuscuta (tusizi)
Deer antler gelatin (lujiaojiao)
Tortoise shell gelatin (guibanjiao)
Achyranthes (niuxi)

    The first three ingredients belong to the yin nourishing portion of Rehmannia Six Formula (Liuwei Dihuang Wan), where rehmannia and cornus nourish the liver and kidney yin and dioscorea nourishes the spleen and kidney yin. Further, both formulas contain lycium fruit and cuscuta. In the modern texts, lycium fruit is known as a yin and blood tonic, while cuscuta is known as a yang tonic and astringent, but cuscuta is also considered somewhat yin nourishing. Cuscuta is commonly paired with lycium fruit to nourish the kidney and liver and benefit vision. Also, both formulas contain deer antler gelatin derived from boiling the antler (described further below). Chinese doctors regard the whole antler as primarily a revitalizing yang tonic with some yin nourishing qualities, while the gelatin is considered to be a milder yang tonic, with greater emphasis on nourishing yin, in a manner similar to tortoise shell (which lacks yang tonic properties). Both tang-kuei (in Yougui Wan) and achyranthes (in Zuogui Wan) are used to nourish the blood and invigorate blood circulation. But, whereas Zuogui Wan incorporates the cooling tortoise shell gelatin, Yougui Wan has the yang-benefiting eucommia and two herbs to warm the kidney yang: cinnamon bark and aconite. These are the same herbs used in Rehmannia Eight Formula (Bawei Dihuang Wan), along with rehmannia, cornus, and dioscorea. So, both of Zhang Jingyue's formulas nourish the kidney yin and essence, and both nourish yang, but Yougui Wan also warms the kidney and invigorates yang. To further emphasize yang tonification, deer antler may be used in place of the gelatin in Yougui Wan.

Because of the rather late introduction of antler in standard traditional Chinese medicine formulations, this ingredient rarely appears in Japanese preparations. The last major influence on Kampo from China was Gong Tingxian (1522-1619) with his book Wanbing Huichun (1587). He did not emphasize kidney tonic strategies. As a result, the **Kampo** literature doesn't reveal antler-based formulas.

During the Qing Dynasty (1644-1910), the use of ginseng and deer antler became quite popular as a method of therapy, sometimes referred to as warm tonic. The Qing Dynasty medical commentator Xu Dachun (1693-1773) complained about over-reliance on these remedies.

Those physicians who prefer to be fashionable use only rapidly supplementing acrid and hot substances, namely ginseng, aconite, dry ginger, red atractylodes, deer antler, and cooked rehmannia. And no matter whether a patient was harmed by cold, heat, or dampness, these physicians go back and forth between these few herbs to compose their prescriptions. Often enough, these herbs are contraindicated in the case of the illness to be treated, and every trial is bound to kill someone. Still, there is not the slightest self-reproach.

Well, this has its origin in the physicians of today who prefer to make lofty speeches to deceive the people. Also, people are pleased if one uses warm and supplementing herbs, and this applies, in particular, to the rich and noble. Those physicians who do not follow these preferences of their patients will not be able to continue their profession for long! Hence, people strive to achieve the best effects, but they cause only unending calamity.

The acrid herbs were dry ginger, aconite, and red atractylodes (which was used at that time as we now use white atractylodes), and all the herbs mentioned were warming, some of them considered hot (though today, all are classified as warm except dry ginger and raw aconite, but not processed aconite). These invigorating tonics were expected to cause people to feel an immediate response to the therapy-a stimulation of their basic energy-compared to the usual tonic approach which might require weeks of regular use of the herbs and a nearly imperceptible daily improvement. Some of these herbs, like ginseng and deer antler, were rare and costly, so the rich sought them out, figuring that they had unique access to important remedies. It is much the same today: many people seek quick fixes and may be drawn to the unusual costly herbs if they can afford them.

Xu argued that reliance on a few popular and quick acting agents tends to be contrary to the most widely accepted methodology, which is to perform differential diagnosis and then prescribe according to need, regardless of the ordinary nature of some herbs or their lack of contemporary popularity. Hence, these warm tonic agents might be contraindicated in cases of heat syndrome, damp-heat, blood heat, stomach fire, phlegm-heat in the lungs, and yin deficiency leading to excess yang. There was much concern during his time about killing patients with wrong prescriptions. Working in the absence of modern medicine, the remedies were used for people with fatal diseases who would die if not cured, and who might be worsened by some of the therapies (for example, raw aconite could be quite toxic if not cooked properly in making a tea). These specific concerns aside, all of the herbs mentioned were recognized as valuable, so long as they were given according to need.

The use of deer antler continued through the Qing Dynasty at a modest level until the 20th century, when it became the subject of modern research methods. Both the Russians (who had been farming deer antler since the 1840s) and the Chinese started subjecting deer antler to analysis by scientific methods, though those methods were relatively crude. About the same time, patent medicine factories sprung up in China and helped fill the growing demand for tonics made with rare ingredients such as deer antler and ginseng. Chinese patent medicine factories now use more than 1,000 kg of deer antler each year. This increased interest and distribution, in turn, led to rapid build-up in the number and size of deer farms.

Species of deer

Initially, antler was collected from several species of wild deer (animals of the Cervidae family). There are 45 species of deer in the world, divided into 17 genera; not all of them have antlers. Two species of deer have been the common source of domestic deer antler for Chinese medicine: Cervus nippon, the sika deer, and Cervus elaphus, the red deer.

The sika deer is an East Asian species, ranging from Vietnam to Taiwan in the south and from China to Korea and Japan in the north; there are about 13 different subspecies of this deer. The sika deer mainly lives in open woodlands and is typically a chestnut red to yellowish brown with white spots on the sides and a dark stripe extending from neck to tail. Sika deer have been introduced to New Zealand for deer farming to produce antlers, and have also been introduced into Europe.

The red deer originally ranged from Europe to Asia, and it has been introduced into New Zealand, Australia, Chile, and Argentina for the purpose of deer farming to produce antler. It has a glossy reddish brown color in summer (but in winter turns drab grey-brown). Red deer prefer open, grassy glades in the forest.

Deer farming

Deer farming has become a huge enterprise outside the Orient. The animal meat is used as food, and the antlers are usually exported to the Orient, though there is a new industry in making antler-based health products for domestic consumption in Canada and other countries. The table on the next page indicates the extent of deer farming.

In Korea, the biggest consumer nation for deer antler, data from the end of 1992 indicated that 143,000 deer were held in pens (about 20 deer each), producing about 100 tons of fresh antler, which yields about 30 tons of dried product. That same year, about three times as much was imported, mainly from New Zealand, Russia, and China. China later became an antler importer rather than exporter, except for finished medicinal preparations and small supplies sent to oversea Chinese pharmacies.

The primary material collected at the deer farms is called velvet. The term originally arose from the fine hairs on the antler, but is now used specifically to indicate the antler's stage of growth: before it calcifies (ossifies). In nature, antlers will fall off after they have ossified; thus, collecting fallen antler doesn't provide the desired "velvet." The older material is still valued: it is boiled to yield deer antler gelatin (described below) and used for certain applications, such as dispersing swellings.

Deer velvet is removed while the deer is under local anesthetic (which is a new practice in China and is a mandated practice in other countries that developed deer antler farming more recently). The antlers then grow back. Alternatively, if the deer is killed for use as food, the antlers are removed afterward. The cut antlers are bathed in boiling water and air dried, and then further dried in the shade or by low temperature baking. The fine hairs may be removed before additional processing. A typical dried antler from the sika deer weighs about 150 grams.

Antler preperations

Traditionally, deer antler is sliced very thinly or ground to powder. It is not commonly boiled in decoctions with herbs because the gelatins easily stick to the herb dregs or cooking pot, and so the loss of valuable material is considered too great. Therefore, the herb powder is usually taken separately.

To make gelatin, ossified antlers (which are less expensive than velvet) are boiled for several hours to release the gelatin (protein components) from the hard matrix. Then, the antler gelatin can be added to an herbal decoction after all the boiling is done and the dregs have been strained. Or, it too can be ground to powder, and consumed directly. After removing the gelatin from the antler, the residual hard antler material is dried and ground up to make lujiaoshuang (degelatinized deer antler), which is mostly used for topical applications (treating boils, eczema, and skin ulcers, serving as an astringent and aid to faster healing). It is also considered of some limited value as a kidney yang tonic if taken at high enough dosage.

Antler pills are a common patent medicine product; the antler is not used alone, but in various formulations. These include liquids in glass vials (ginseng-deer antler, similar to the ginseng-royal jelly product; there is a combination with ginseng, antler, and royal jelly); pills used as sexual tonics (antler combined with epimedium, cynomorium, ginseng, and lycium fruit); and general tonics (complex formulas with herbs for tonifying qi and yang, and nourishing yin and blood).

The thin slices are made by removing the outer, hairy portion of the antler, soaking the antler in hot alcohol to soften it, and then carefully slicing it to produce round wafers. The slices are best suited for soaking in wine to make a "tincture" of antler, sometimes referred to as pantocrin (or pantocrine), based on the Russian designation for the alcohol extract. Very thin slices (virtually clear) **can be eaten directly.**

Antler constitutes

Antler is a simple extension of bone, so it has a calcium-phosphate matrix of hydroxyapatite, $Ca_{10}(PO_4)_6(OH)_2$, integrated with smaller amounts of calcium carbonate ($CaCO_3$); its composition is similar to that of human bones. Thus, one of the therapeutic roles of taking deer antler is as a source of calcium to help prevent or treat osteoporosis, which is consistent with the traditional bone strengthening action of deer antler. An analysis of the ossified antler showed that 73% is hydroxyapatite and related mineral compounds, while 27% is organic materials. If consumed as a powder (rather than a decoction), a person taking 3 grams of deer antler (see dosage section, below) will get about 800 mg of calcium. Hydroxyapatite is considered one of the most efficiently absorbed forms of calcium available. In velvet, the hydroxyapatite is about 50%, so the calcium in 3 grams is about 600 mg.

Deer antler also has a substantial amount of gelatinous components, ones that have become widely publicized in recent years, though from other source materials: glucosamine sulfate, chondroitin sulfate (which is a polymer of glucosamine), and collagen. These compounds have been shown to benefit the joints in cases of osteoarthritis by providing substrate materials useful for regenerating the body's connective tissues (collagen) found in joints and sinews. In addition, they may have some anti-inflammatory action, useful for arthritis and tendinitis. These actions of the gelatin portion support the traditional concept that antler benefits joints and ligaments. In a 3-gram dose of ossified deer antler powder, one will obtain about 750 mg of these substances, which is low compared to therapeutic amounts taken as supplements for osteoarthritis (about 1,500 mg/day); 3 grams of velvet antler will provide the desired 1,500 mg. If deer antler gelatin is consumed, there is an even higher proportion of these ingredients, though some of the components may be transformed during the prolonged boiling into less active forms, so the dosage of gelatin to use is higher than for antler velvet.

Recently, the traditional use of antler to nourish the bone marrow and blood has been validated by studies in which the active components responsible were identified: monoacetyldiglycerides (9, 10). These are small molecules that stimulate the marrow stem cells that produce blood cells (see illustration, next page; 11). Inhibition of hematopoiesis (blood cell production) occurs with several cancer drugs and with radiation therapy; some disease processes, such as myelodysplastic syndrome (MDS), involve progressive decline in stem cell activity with undetermined causes. If further research confirms the therapeutic importance of the monoacetyldiglycerides, they can be synthesized in large quantity. In the meantime, deer antler is the main therapeutic source for them (the amount present in antler has not been quantified).

Stem cells leading to various blood lines. The basic marrow stem cell differentiates during early fetal development into two types of stem cells, the lymphoid (which produces lymphocytes) and the myeloid (which produces all the other blood cells). Platelets (thrombocytes) are not true blood cells, but are cytoplasmic fragments of the megakaryocytes. T-cells are lymphoid cells that differentiate via action of the thymus gland. All the cell lines except erythrocytes (red blood cells) and megakaryocytes are involved with immune responses. Thus, deer antler, when used to stimulate the stem cells in patients with bone marrow depression, may improve immune responses, as indicated by laboratory animal studies.

Deer antler also has essential fatty acids, making up about 2.5% of the velvet antler (not enough to be clinically active) and insulin-dependent growth factor (for which it is not known whether there is any clinical effect). Other organic compounds have been detected, but in miniscule amounts.

Dosage

The velvet antler in powdered form is typically used in dosages of 1-3 grams/day. Less than 3 grams may be a low dosage for promoting bone marrow function; the dosage levels traditionally indicated may reflect the rarity and expense of the antler (which is now partly alleviated by the increase in deer farming, but velvet is still relatively costly). The 3-gram dosage is probably essential for hematopoietic effect and for benefitting joints and tendons.

Antler gelatin, because it is obtained from older antler material, is relatively inexpensive, is milder, and is used in larger quantities, 6-9 grams. De-gelatinized antler is consumed in dosages of 6-9 grams, or more.

Traditional Medicine Commentaries

The book Ten Lectures on the Use of Medicinals from the Personal Experience of Jiao Shude provides these insights:

Lurong (velvet deer antler): Warm in nature and sweet and salty in flavor, lurong supplements kidney yang, strengthens sinew and bone, boosts sinew and marrow, and nourishes the blood. It is used for patterns of vacuity detriment, such a kidney deficiency and cold limbs, soreness of the limbs, dizzy head and blurred vision, seminal emission, and impotence.

Lujiao (ossified deer antler): Salty in flavor and warm in nature, lujiao supplements kidney yang and boosts essence and blood. It is similar in action to, and can substitute for, lurong, but it is less effective.

Lujiaojiao (deer antler gelatin): Sweet in flavor and warm in nature, lujiaojiao warms and supplements the kidney, supplements yang within yin, frees the blood of the thoroughfare vessel (chongmai), engenders essence and blood, and stanches flooding (excessive uterine bleeding)….It is mostly used for flooding and spotting, vaginal discharge, deficiency bleeding, and yin type flat-abscess (lumps that are not red, swollen, hot, or painful).

Comparisons: Lurong is commonly used as a drastic liver-kidney supplementing medicinal. It has greater supplementing power than lujiao. Lujiao, by contrast, has a moderate liver-kidney supplementing effect, but it quickens the blood, dissipates stasis, and disperses swelling and toxin with greater strength than lurong….Used processed or as a glue (lujiaojiao), it tends to warm and supplement the liver and kidney, enrich and nourish essence-blood. Lujiaojiao is similar in action to lurong, but being slower to supplement, it must be taken over a long period of time to be effective. Lujiaoshuang, which is the dregs left after making lujiaojiao, is less warming and supplementing than either lujiao or lujiaojiao. Lujiaoshuang is used for spleen-stomach deficiency cold, low food intake, and sloppy stool, and it is also used as a substitute for lujiao and lujiaojiao, in which case the dosage must be increased.

The problem of "flooding" and spotting was described by Liu Yiren in his book Heart Transmission of Medicine (ca. 1850; 13).

The disease of flooding and leaking is due to detriment of the chong (penetrating) and ren (conception) vessels. The chongmai is the sea of blood of the twelve channels, and the renmai is the original qi of engenderment and nourishment. If these two vessels suffer detriment, the blood will consequently move frenetically. At its onset, this disease is categorized as repletion heat, requiring clearing heat. Later on, it is characterized as deficiency heat, requiring nourishing the blood and clearing heat. If it endures for many days, it is categorized as deficiency cold, requiring warming the channels and supplementing the blood.

Although antler wasn't commonly used during Liu Yiren's time, it would today be a primary choice for treating the deficiency cold syndrome that he described. Since bleeding is part of the syndrome, antler gelatin would be utilized, probably with tortoise shell.

The Advanced Textbook of Traditional Chinese Medicine and Pharmacology (14) notes the main uses for deer antler (lurong):

a) Chronic diseases marked by general lassitude and spiritlessness, lumbago, and cold limbs, polyuria with clear urine, impotence, spermatorrhea, and leukorrhagia with clear discharge, for which it is often used with cooked rehmannia, eucommia, and cistanche.

b) Infantile maldevelopment marked by weakness of the muscles and bones, incomplete closure of the fontanel, and retarded speech and movement, for which it is often combined with cooked rehmannia and cornus [it is sometimes added to Rehmannia Six Formula, which has these ingredients, and which was designed for promoting healthy growth of children who displayed slow development].

c) Chronic diseases with blood deficiency and liver and kidney deficiency, for which it is often used with ginseng, astragalus, cooked rehmannia, and tang-kuei.

d) Deficiency of the extra meridians (e.g., chongmai) with incessant uterine bleeding, for which it is often prescribed with gelatin, sepia bone, tang-kuei, and tortoise shell.

The effects of lujiao, lujiaojiao, and lujiaoshuang derived from the antlers are basically the same: warming and nourishing kidney yang. But, lujiao also activates blood circulation and relieves swelling, lujiaojiao is more effective for nourishing blood and checking bleeding, and lujiaoshuang possesses an astringent effect (i.e., for incontinence of urine, uterine bleeding, and leukorrhea).

References

1. Yang Shouzhong (translator), The Divine Farmer's Materia Medica, 1998 Blue Poppy Press, Boulder, CO.

2. Huang Bingshan and Wang Yuxia, Thousand Formulas and Thousand Herbs of Traditional Chinese Medicine, volume 2, 1993 Heilongjiang Education Press, Harbin.

3. Unschuld PU, Forgotten Traditions of Ancient Chinese Medicine, 1990 Paradigm Publications, Brookline, MA.

4. Anonymous, History of Deer Farming, The Deer Farmer, http://www.deerfarmer.co.nz/ihistory.htm, WHAM Media Ltd., New Zealand.

5. Guo Yinfeng, et al., Sustainability of Wildlife Use in Traditional Chinese Medicine, in Conserving China's Biodiversity (MacKinnon J, et al., editors) 1996 China Environmental Science Press. Beijing. pp. 190-221.

6. Ministry of Agriculture and Forestry, New Zealand, Dynamics of supply and demand for New Zealand venison and velvet, 1994; http://www.maf.govt.nz/mafnet/rural-nz/

7. Mkukuma LD, et al., The relationship between mineral content and mineral composition,

University of Aberdeen Department of Orthopaedic Surgery, http://www.abdn.ac.uk/orthopaedics/bone_mineral_res.htm

8. Marshal LA, Velvet antler under the microscope, Nutrition Science News 2000; http://www.newhope.com/nutritionsciencenews/NSN_backs/Mar_00/velvet.cfm

9. Yang HO, et al., Purification and structural determination of hematopoietic stem cell-stimulating monoacetyldiglycerides from Cervus nippon (deer antler), Chemical and Pharmaceutical Bulletin 2004; 52(7): 874-878.

10. Yang HO, et al., Stimulatory effects of monoacetyldiglycerides on hematopoiesis, Biology and Pharmacology Bulletin 2004; 27(7): 1121-1125.

11. University of Arizona, Biology Project: http://www.biology.arizona.edu/

12. Mitchell C, et al. (translators), Ten Lectures on the Use of Medicinals from the Personal Experience of Jiao Shude, 2003 Paradigm Publications, Brookline, MA.

13. Yang Shouzhong (translator), The Heart Transmission of Medicine, 1997 Blue Poppy Press, Boulder, CO.

14. State Administration of Traditional Chinese Medicine, Advanced Textbook on Traditional Chinese Medicine and Pharmacology, (volume. 2).